Foundations of Developmental Care

Guest Editors

JOY V. BROWNE, PhD, PCNS-BC
ROBERT D. WHITE, MD

CLINICS IN PERINATOLOGY

www.perinatology.theclinics.com

Consulting Editor

LUCKY JAIN, MD, MBA

December 2011 • Volume 38 • Number 4

SAUNDERS an imprint of ELSEVIER, Inc.

W.B. SAUNDERS COMPANY
A Division of Elsevier Inc.

Elsevier, Inc. ● 1600 John F. Kennedy Blvd. ● Suite 1800 ● Philadelphia, PA 19103-2899

http://www.theclinics.com

CLINICS IN PERINATOLOGY Volume 38, Number 4
December 2011 ISSN 0095-5108, ISBN-13: 978-1-4557-1119-2

Editor: Kerry Holland
Developmental Editor: Donald Mumford

Clinics in Perinatology (ISSN 0095-5108) is published quarterly by Elsevier Inc., 360 Park Avenue South, New York, NY 10010-1710. Months of issue are March, June, September, and December. Business and Editorial Offices: 1600 John F. Kennedy Blvd., Ste. 1800, Philadelphia, PA 19103-2899. Customer Service Office: 3251 Riverport Lane, Maryland Heights, MO 63043. Periodicals postage paid at New York, NY and additional mailing offices. Subscription prices are $273.00 per year (US individuals), $401.00 per year (US institutions), $326.00 per year (Canadian individuals), $509.00 per year (Canadian institutions), $400.00 per year (foreign individuals), $509.00 per year (foreign institutions), $130.00 per year (US students), and $187.00 per year (Canadian and foreign students). Foreign air speed delivery is included in all Clinics subscription prices. All prices are subject to change without notice. **POSTMASTER:** Send address changes to *Clinics in Perinatology*, Elsevier Health Sciences Division, Subscription Customer Service, 3251 Riverport Lane, Maryland Heights, MO 63043. **Customer Service: Telephone: 1-800-654-2452** (U.S. and Canada); **1-314-447-8871** (outside U.S. and Canada). **Fax: 1-314-447-8029. E-mail: journalscustomerservice-usa@elsevier.com** (for print support); **journalsonlinesupport-usa@elsevier.com** (for online support).

Reprints. For copies of 100 or more, of articles in this publication, please contact the Commercial Reprints Department, Elsevier Inc., 360 Park Avenue South, New York, NY 10010-1710. Tel. (212) 633-3812; Fax: (212) 482-1935; email: reprints@elsevier.com.

Clinics in Perinatology is also pubilshed in Spanish by McGraw-Hill Interamericana Editores S.A., P.O. Box 5-237, 06500 Mexico D.F., Mexico.

Clinics in Perinatology is covered in *MEDLINE/PubMed (Index Medicus) Current Contents, Excepta Medica, BIOSIS and ISI/BIOMED.*

Printed in the United States of America.

Contributors

CONSULTING EDITOR

LUCKY JAIN, MD, MBA
Richard Blumberg Professor and Executive Vice Chairman, Department of Pediatrics, Emory University School of Medicine, Atlanta, Georgia

GUEST EDITORS

JOY V. BROWNE, PhD, PCNS-BC
Clinical Professor of Pediatrics and Psychiatry, JFK Partners Center for Family and Infant Interaction, University of Colorado Anschutz Medical Campus, Aurora, Colorado; Professor, School of Nursing and Midwifery, Queen's University of Belfast, Belfast, Northern Ireland

ROBERT D. WHITE, MD
Clinical Assistant Professor Pediatrics, Indiana University School of Medicine; Adjunct Assistant Professor of Psychology, University of Notre Dame; and Director, Regional Newborn Program, Pediatrix Medical Group, Memorial Hospital, South Bend, Indiana

AUTHORS

KATHARINA BRAUN, PhD
Director, and Professor of Zoology and Developmental Neurobiology, Department of Zoology and Developmental Neurobiology, Institute of Biology, Otto von Guericke University Magdeburg, Magdeburg, Germany

JOY V. BROWNE, PhD, PCNS-BC
Clinical Professor of Pediatrics and Psychiatry, JFK Partners Center for Family and Infant Interaction, University of Colorado Anschutz Medical Campus, Aurora, Colorado; Professor, School of Nursing and Midwifery, Queen's University of Belfast, Belfast, Northern Ireland

NINA BURTCHEN, MSc
Division of Developmental Neuroscience, Department of Psychiatry, Columbia University, New York, New York

FRANCES A. CHAMPAGNE, PhD
Assistant Professor, Department of Psychology, Columbia University, New York, New York

JOHN L. DRYSDALE, BAppSc(Phty) Hons
Senior Physiotherapist (Paediatrics), and Research Associate, Neuromotor Plasticity and Development, DX 650-517 Robinson Institute, Discipline of Obstetrics and Gynaecology, School of Paediatrics and Reproductive Health, University of Adelaide, Adelaide, Australia

STANLEY N. GRAVEN, MD
Professor, Department of Community and Family Health, College of Public Health, University of South Florida, Tampa, Florida

KATHRYN M.A. GUDSNUK
Department of Psychology, Columbia University, New York, New York

LUCKY JAIN, MD, MBA
Richard Blumberg Professor and Executive Vice Chairman, Department of Pediatrics, Emory University School of Medicine, Atlanta, Georgia

KARINE KLEINHAUS, MD, MPH
Departments of Psychiatry and Environmental Medicine, New York University School of Medicine, New York University, New York, New York

ROBERT LICKLITER, PhD
Professor, Department of Psychology, Infant Development Research Center, Florida International University, Miami, Florida

SARAH V. LIPCHOCK, PhD
Postdoctoral Fellow, Monell Chemical Senses Center, Philadelphia, Pennsylvania

JULIE A. MENNELLA, PhD
Member, Monell Chemical Senses Center, Philadelphia, Pennsylvania

CHRISTINE MOON, PhD
Department of Psychology, Pacific Lutheran University, Tacoma, Washington

JULIE A. OWENS, PhD
Professor of Obstetrics and Gynaecology, Research Centre for the Early Origins of Health and Disease, DX 650-521 Robinson Institute, Discipline of Obstetrics and Gynaecology, School of Paediatrics and Reproductive Health, University of Adelaide, Adelaide, Australia

ROSEMARIE PERRY, BS
Emotional Brain Institute, The Nathan S. Kline Institute for Psychiatric Research, Child and Adolescent Psychiatry; Sackler Graduate Program, Sackler Institute, New York University School of Medicine, New York, New York

JULIA B. PITCHER, PhD
M.S. McLeod Research Fellow (Paediatric Medicine), Neuromotor Plasticity and Development, DX 650-517 Robinson Institute, Discipline of Obstetrics and Gynaecology, School of Paediatrics and Reproductive Health, University of Adelaide, Adelaide, Australia

DANIELLE R. REED, PhD
Member, Monell Chemical Senses Center, Philadelphia, Pennsylvania

MICHAEL C. RIDDING, PhD
Associate Professor, National Health and Medical Research Council; Senior Research Fellow, Neuromotor Plasticity and Development, DX 650-517 Robinson Institute, Discipline of Obstetrics and Gynaecology, School of Paediatrics and Reproductive Health, University of Adelaide, Adelaide, Australia

ERIN SUNDSETH ROSS, PhD, CCC-SLP
Clinical Instructor of Pediatrics, JFK Partners Center for Family and Infant Interaction, University of Colorado Anschutz Medical Campus, Aurora, Colorado

LUKE A. SCHNEIDER, PhD
Postdoctoral Research Associate, Neuromotor Plasticity and Development, DX 650-517
Robinson Institute, Discipline of Obstetrics and Gynaecology, School of Paediatrics and
Reproductive Health, University of Adelaide, Adelaide, Australia

ALIZA SLOAN, MA
Emotional Brain Institute, The Nathan S. Kline Institute for Psychiatric Research, Child and
Adolescent Psychiatry, New York University School of Medicine, New York, New York

REGINA SULLIVAN, PhD
Emotional Brain Institute, The Nathan S. Kline Institute for Psychiatric Research, Child and
Adolescent Psychiatry, New York University School of Medicine, New York, New York

ROBERT D. WHITE, MD
Clinical Assistant Professor Pediatrics, Indiana University School of Medicine; Adjunct
Assistant Professor of Psychology, University of Notre Dame; and Director, Regional
Newborn Program, Pediatrix Medical Group, Memorial Hospital, South Bend, Indiana

Contents

> Early life infant-caregiver attachment is a dynamic, bidirectional process
> that involving both the infant and caregiver. Infant attachment appears
> to have a dual function. First, it ensures the infant remains close to the
> caregiver in order to receive necessary care for survival. Second, the qual-
> ity of attachment and its associated sensory stimuli organize the brain to
> define the infant's cognitive and emotional development. Here we present
> attachment within an historical view and highlight the importance of inte-
> grating human and animal research in understanding infant care.

> Auditory perception and learning take place during the third trimester of ges-
> tation. Fetuses and newborns who lack typical auditory experience can go on
> to develop typical socioemotional attachment and language, given a support-
> ive environment. For hospitalized preterm infants in developmentally
> sensitive neonatal intensive care units, detrimental effects of deviant early au-
> ditory experience may be remediated by later experience, but much is un-
> known about the causes of language deficits of prematurity. Prenatal
> auditory stimulation programs that incorporate audio speakers against the
> maternal belly should be discouraged because of possible overstimulation
> effects on the developing auditory system and sleep/wake state organization.

> Much of the early development of the human visual system occurs while
> the preterm infant is in the neonatal intensive care unit (NICU). Critical
> events and processes happen between 20 and 40 weeks' gestational
> age, before the onset of vision at term birth. Knowledge of the develop-
> ment of the visual system and the timing of the processes involved is
> essential to adapting NICU care to support all neurosensory development
> including visual development.

> The knowledge that neonatal emotional experience and associated learn-
> ing processes are critical in the maturation of prefronto-limbic circuits
> emphasizes the importance of preterm and neonatal care. The further
> improvement of care and intervention strategies requires a deeper under-
> standing of epigenetic mechanisms mediating experience-induced synap-
> tic reorganization underlying the emergence of emotional and cognitive
> behavioral traits. Interdisciplinary research efforts are needed in which
> pediatricians and developmental biologists and psychologists merge their
> knowledge, concepts, and methodology. The hope is that the translational
> relevance of research efforts can be improved through a greater interac-
> tion between basic and clinical scientists.

Kathryn M.A. Gudsnuk and Frances A. Champagne

Early-life adversity can affect brain development and behavior. Emerging evidence from studies on both humans and rodents suggests that epigenetic mechanisms may play a critical role in shaping our biology in response to the quality of the environment. This article highlights the research findings suggesting that prenatal maternal stress, postnatal maternal care, and infant neglect/abuse can lead to epigenetic variation, which may have long-term effects on stress responsivity, neuronal plasticity, and behavior.

Joy V. Browne

Neonatology has optimized medical outcomes for high-risk newborns yet neurodevelopmental outcomes continue to be a concern. Basic science, clinical research, and environmental design perspectives have shown the impact of the caregiving environment on the developing brain and the role of professional caregivers in providing supportive intervention to both infants and their families. This recognition has prompted a focus on early developmentally supportive care (DSC) for high-risk newborns both in the hospital and in community follow up. DSC has emerged as a recognized standard of care in most neonatal intensive care units. Still, many questions remain and much integrative research is needed.

Joy V. Browne and Erin Sundseth Ross

Many high-risk and preterm infants have difficulty with successful feeding and subsequent optimal growth during their stay in the neonatal intensive care unit as well as in the months after discharge. Environmental, procedural, and medical issues necessary for treatment of the hospitalized infant present challenges for the development of successful eating skills. Emerging data describe eating as a predictable neurodevelopmental process that depends on the infant's organization of physiologic processes, motor tone and movement, level of arousal, and ability to simultaneously regulate these processes.

Robert D. White

The environment of care has been recognized as an important factor in the healing process for centuries. This is true for all individuals but none more so than newborn infants, for whom the hospital is not only a place of healing but also where an extraordinary and unique period of growth and development must occur—it cannot wait until after the infant is well and discharged home. This article describes the optimal environment for developmental care in the neonatal intensive care unit.

GOAL STATEMENT

The goal of *Clinics in Perinatology* is to keep practicing neonatologists and maternal-fetal medicine specialists up to date with current clinical practice in perinatology by providing timely articles reviewing the state of the art in patient care.

ACCREDITATION

The *Clinics in Perinatology* is planned and implemented in accordance with the Essential Areas and Policies of the Accreditation Council for Continuing Medical Education (ACCME) through the joint sponsorship of the University of Virginia School of Medicine and Elsevier. The University of Virginia School of Medicine is accredited by the ACCME to provide continuing medical education for physicians.

The University of Virginia School of Medicine designates this enduring material activity for a maximum of 15 *AMA PRA Category 1 Credit*(s)™ for each issue, 60 credits per year. Physicians should only claim credit commensurate with the extent of their participation in the activity.

The American Medical Association has determined that physicians not licensed in the US who participate in this CME enduring material activity are eligible for a maximum of 15 *AMA PRA Category 1 Credit*(s)™ for each issue, 60 credits per year.

Credit can be earned by reading the text material, taking the CME examination online at http://www.theclinics.com/home/cme, and completing the evaluation. After taking the test, you will be required to review any and all incorrect answers. Following completion of the test and evaluation, your credit will be awarded and you may print your certificate.

FACULTY DISCLOSURE/CONFLICT OF INTEREST

The University of Virginia School of Medicine, as an ACCME accredited provider, endorses and strives to comply with the Accreditation Council for Continuing Medical Education (ACCME) Standards of Commercial Support, Commonwealth of Virginia statutes, University of Virginia policies and procedures, and associated federal and private regulations and guidelines on the need for disclosure and monitoring of proprietary and financial interests that may affect the scientific integrity and balance of content delivered in continuing medical education activities under our auspices.

The University of Virginia School of Medicine requires that all CME activities accredited through this institution be developed independently and be scientifically rigorous, balanced and objective in the presentation/discussion of its content, theories and practices.

All authors/editors participating in an accredited CME activity are expected to disclose to the readers relevant financial relationships with commercial entities occurring within the past 12 months (such as grants or research support, employee, consultant, stock holder, member of speakers bureau, etc.). The University of Virginia School of Medicine will employ appropriate mechanisms to resolve potential conflicts of interest to maintain the standards of fair and balanced education to the reader. Questions about specific strategies can be directed to the Office of Continuing Medical Education, University of Virginia School of Medicine, Charlottesville, Virginia.

The faculty and staff of the University of Virginia Office of Continuing Medical Education have no financial affiliations to disclose.

The authors/editors listed below have identified no professional or financial affiliations for themselves or their spouse/partner:

Robert Boyle, MD (Test Author); Katharina Braun, PhD; Joy V. Browne, PhD, PCNS-BC (Guest Editor); Nina Burtchen, MD, MSc; Frances A. Champagne, PhD; John L. Drysdale, BAppSc(Phty) Hons; Stanley N. Graven, MD; Kathryn M.A. Gudsnuk; Kerry Holland, (Acquisitions Editor); Lucky Jain, MD, MBA (Consulting Editor); Karine Kleinhaus, MD, MPH; Robert Lickliter, PhD; Sarah V. Lipchock, PhD; Julie A. Mennella, PhD; Christine Moon, PhD; Julie A. Owens, PhD; Rosemarie Perry, BS; Julia B. Pitcher, PhD; Danielle R. Reed, PhD; Michael C. Ridding, PhD; Luke A. Schneider, PhD; Aliza Sloan, MA; Regina Sullivan, PhD; and Robert D. White, MD (Guest Editor).

The authors/editors listed below identified the following professional or financial affiliations for themselves or their spouse/partner:

Erin Sundseth Ross, PhD, CCC-SLP is a consultant for Nestec, a division of Nestle.

Disclosure of Discussion of Non-FDA Approved Uses for Pharmaceutical Products and/or Medical Devices

The University of Virginia School of Medicine, as an ACCME provider, requires that all faculty presenters identify and disclose any off-label uses for pharmaceutical and medical device products. The University of Virginia School of Medicine recommends that each physician fully review all the available data on new products or procedures prior to clinical use.

TO ENROLL

To enroll in the Clinics in Perinatology Continuing Medical Education program, call customer service at 1-800-654-2452 or visit us online at www.theclinics.com/home/cme. The CME program is available to subscribers for an additional fee of $196.00.

THE CLINICS ARE NOW AVAILABLE ONLINE!

Access your subscription at:
www.theclinics.com

Foreword

The Foundations of Newborn Brain Development

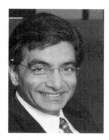

Lucky Jain, MD, MBA
Consulting Editor

In a recent article published in the magazine *New Yorker* entitled, "A Child in Time," Jerome Groopman[1] captures the journey of a prematurely born infant into adulthood and cites the many advances that have helped secure a better future for the tiniest of preterm infants. The caption accompanying a picture on the front page aptly reads, "Recent advances have boosted parents' hopes, but uncertainties remain." Indeed, a day in a high-risk developmental follow-up clinic examining these growing infants will reveal the broad spectrum of outcomes that await them—from frank cerebral palsy to a brilliant young child completely unaware of the close scare of preterm birth.

Questions remain though: why do two neonates with seemingly similar anatomical injury have such different outcomes? Why are different parts of the brain, and the diverse functions they control, impacted so differently by the same pathologic process? This issue of the *Clinics in Perinatology* makes a serious attempt to bridge the gaps in our knowledge of what makes the developing brain so vulnerable and what can be done to optimize its outcome. Drs Browne and White are to be congratulated for having put together a superb volume of articles that lays the foundation for appropriate developmental care.

Questions also remain about the impact of the rapidly changing social environment on the growing brain. Early childhood developmental experiences such as lack of breast feeding, absence of a consistent mother figure, repeated painful stimuli, and lack of circadian rhythms (to name a few) may have long-term implications that have not been fully elucidated. The picture is further muddied by the complex social environment we now live in with an ever-increasing opportunity for maladaptation. This is particularly important for the child with borderline deficits, who runs the risk of alienation from siblings and peers because of being unable to keep up with the technology that surrounds us. Some of these maladaptation issues can manifest much later in life as we have learned from the few longitudinal cohorts that we currently have access to.

Clin Perinatol 38 (2011) xiii–xiv
doi:10.1016/j.clp.2011.10.001   **perinatology.theclinics.com**
0095-5108/11/$ – see front matter © 2011 Elsevier Inc. All rights reserved.

One such recent report shows higher mortality in the third decade of life for infants born even slightly preterm.[2] Another report from the same cohort shows a higher risk of adverse neurological outcomes in infants born at late preterm gestation.[3]

Finally, the growing brain and body are deceptively capable of keeping adverse effects masked until cognitive and motor functions can be meaningfully tested. This puts a great burden on the busy front-line pediatrician to detect and address subtle signs of disability. And yet, for the many trainees who are gearing up to populate the next generation of front-line providers, preoccupation with lab values and count-less levels of documentation leave little time to learn the art of conducting a thorough neurologic exam. It is our hope that optimizing developmental outcomes will remain a rigorous focus for all providers, just as improving survival and early outcomes has been over the years.

Lucky Jain, MD, MBA
Department of Pediatrics
Emory University School of Medicine
2015 Uppergate Drive
Atlanta, GA 30322, USA

E-mail address:
ljain@emory.edu

REFERENCES

1. Groopman J. A child in time. The New Yorker October 24, 2011;1–7.
2. Crump C, Sundquist K, Sundquist J, et al. Gestational age at birth and mortality in young adulthood. JAMA 2011;306:1233–40.
3. Lindstrom K, Winbladh B, Haglund B, et al. Preterm infants as young adults: a Swedish national cohort study. Pediatrics 2007;120:70–7.

Preface

Foundations of Developmental Care

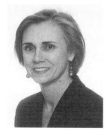
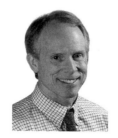

Joy V. Browne, PhD, PCNS-BC   Robert D. White, MD
Guest Editors

Advances in neonatal care have led to better survival for high-risk newborns, but serious questions remain regarding neurodevelopmental outcomes. The impact on the developing brain of the physical, care-giving, and family environments has received growing attention. In large part, the catalyst for bringing these research findings into clinical practice came from national meetings and study groups of scientists, clinicians, administrators, and architects headed by Dr Stanley Graven.[1,2]

This volume is designed to aggregate current thinking about neonatal neurodevelopment, thereby helping clinicians understand and apply this knowledge to the developmental challenges of high-risk newborns under intensive care. It recognizes contributions of basic science to our understanding of development from molecular function to neurophysiology to later observable behavior. We highlight two themes that are consistently represented throughout the authors' articles. First, development is continuous from the fetus to the newborn to the older infant. Fetal learning is essential for attachment to the mother and to assure protection and survival. Infant learning influences not only immediate behavioral organization and long-term developmental outcomes, but perhaps generational epigenetic change as well. Stressful, painful, or nonsupportive experiences likely influence long-term developmental outcomes, potentially to the next generation. However, infants also show resilience in brain development, which has implications for the application of early, individualized, relationship-based intervention from fetal to newborn to growing infant periods. Second, during the continuous developmental process, there are sensitive periods when brain development is particularly malleable and expectant of well-timed, appropriately organized input from the environment. During these sensitive periods, it is essential that the infant, based on his or her specific behaviorally communicated needs, receive the most appropriately organized and timed input from the caregiving environment, and in particular from the mother. Individualized developmental care using the Newborn Individualized Developmental Care and Assessment Program, which includes

Clin Perinatol 38 (2011) xv–xvii
doi:10.1016/j.clp.2011.09.001   **perinatology.theclinics.com**

Kangaroo Mother Care, has provided us with an evidence-based template and strategies for optimizing the experience of the infant during sensitive periods. We also have emerging evidence of the importance of the father in support of infant socioemotional development. Traditional models of care-giving in the newborn intensive care unit must change to encourage this parent–infant contact during sensitive periods of brain development.

We owe many thanks to our developmental psychobiology colleagues, whose research efforts are helping us as clinicians to identify theoretical and neurophysiologic foundations of development so we can apply them to human infants, and, in particular, those who are at high risk for adverse developmental outcomes. We also thank those scientists and architects who have helped change our perspective on environmental design in support of families and their infants under intensive care. Most especially, we thank those who have had the foresight to understand how individualized, relationship-based care for infants and families can change short- and long-term neurodevelopmental outcomes. As Amiel-Tison and Stewart have noted, infants have "one brain for life."[3] With evidence-based, developmentally appropriate intervention, which Als has referred to as "brain care,"[4] we have the opportunity to optimize the structure and function of that one brain and to provide infants and families with the best beginnings possible.

Optimizing neurodevelopmental outcomes of high-risk newborns should, in large part, focus on early nurturing relationships between the mother and father and their baby, and more research should further describe optimal intervention at each developmental period. Newborn intensive care units have an opportunity to become integrated research laboratories where scientists can provide optimal research design, clinicians can provide a pragmatic and safe clinical approach, and environmental design can provide for a nonintimidating, regulating, and nurturing experience for the emerging family.

Joy V. Browne, PhD, PCNS-BC
Departments of Pediatrics and Psychiatry
JFK Partners Center for Family and Infant Interaction
University of Colorado Anschutz Medical Campus
13121 East 17th Avenue
Room L28-5117
Aurora, CO 80045, USA

Robert D. White, MD
Indiana University School of Medicine
University of Notre Dame
Regional Newborn Program
Memorial Hospital
615 North Michigan Street
South Bend, IN 46601, USA

E-mail addresses:
joy.browne@childrenscolorado.org (J.V. Browne)
Robert_White@pediatrix.com (R.D. White)

REFERENCES

1. Graven SN, Bowen FW Jr, Brooten D, et al. The high-risk infant environment. Part 1. The role of the neonatal intensive care unit in the outcome of high-risk infants. J Perinatol 1992;12(2):164–72.
2. Graven SN, Bowen FW Jr, Brooten D, et al. The high-risk infant environment. Part 2. The role of caregiving and the social environment. J Perinatol 1992;12(3):267–75.
3. Amiel Tison C, Stewart A. The newborn infant: one brain for life. Institut Natl Del LA Sante; 1994.
4. Als H. Caring for the preterm infant earliest brain development and experience. International and interdisciplinary symposium: the infant—attachment, neurobiology and genes. Munich (Germany): Hellbrugge Foundation, University of Munich; 2006.

The Integrated Development of Sensory Organization

Robert Lickliter, PhD

KEYWORDS

- Prenatal sensory experience • Neural plasticity
- Sensory integration • Intersensory redundancy

SENSORY INTEGRATION AND ORGANIZATION

Most objects and events present a complex mix of visual, auditory, tactile, and olfactory stimulation to the senses. How do young infants determine which patterns of sensory stimulation belong together and which ones are unrelated? For much of the twentieth century, most developmental scientists assumed that infants must gradually learn to coordinate and integrate information obtained by the separate sensory systems.[1–3] From this view, information had to be integrated across the separate senses through a gradual process of association for infants to perceive unified objects and events. This integration was thought to occur by the infant interacting with objects, experiencing concurrent feedback from different senses, and associating, assimilating, or calibrating one sense to another. For example, the pioneering developmental psychologist Jean Piaget[3,4] proposed that it was not until well into the first half year after birth that vision and touch begin to be integrated. Through acting on objects, tactile feedback was thought to gradually endow the 2-dimensional visual image of an object with 3 dimensionality. The attainment of perceptual abilities such as size and shape constancy, visually guided reaching, and object permanence were thought by Piaget and his colleagues[5] to be slow to emerge and to depend on the gradual development of sensory integration. Before this integration, the visual world of the infant was thought to consist of images shrinking, expanding, changing shape, and disappearing and then reappearing. Until the gradual achievement of sensory integration, infants were thought to perceive unrelated patterns of visual, acoustic, or tactile stimulation, expressed by the well-known description of the world of the newborn infant by William James as a "blooming, buzzing confusion."

The author has nothing to disclose.
The writing of this article was supported by NICHD grant RO1048423 and NSF grant BCS 1057898.

Department of Psychology, Infant Development Research Center, Florida International University, 11200 SW 8th Street, Miami, FL 33199, USA
E-mail address: licklite@fiu.edu

Clin Perinatol 38 (2011) 591–603
doi:10.1016/j.clp.2011.08.007
0095-5108/11/$ – see front matter © 2011 Elsevier Inc. All rights reserved.

perinatology.theclinics.com

Infant-based research performed over the last several decades has seriously challenged this traditional view of early sensory organization and perceptual development. It is now known that the senses function in concert even in very early infancy and that young brains are organized to use the information they derive from the various sensory systems to enhance the likelihood that objects and events will be detected rapidly, identified correctly, and responded to appropriately, even during very early development.[6] Infants are sensitive to audiovisual synchrony from birth. For example, even newborns can match visual with auditory information[7] and orient visually toward a sound.[8] By 4 months of age, infants presented with 2 superimposed films and an audio track that corresponds to only one of the films will attend to the film that is in synchrony with the sound track.[9] Such abilities are likely based on young infants' sensitivity to relatively low levels of intersensory relations, including intensity and temporal synchrony.[10,11]

Evidence obtained from neurophysiologic research over the last decade indicates that the brain is remarkably skilled at integrating input from the different sensory systems to maximize the information available for perception and action.[6,12–14] Further, the ability to integrate information from different senses is not limited to any particular brain structure. Multisensory integration has been found in neurons at many locations in the nervous system, including subcortical areas such as the superior colliculus, early cortical areas such as the primary visual and auditory cortices, and higher cortical levels such as the superior temporal sulcus and intraparietal areas.[13,15–17] Available evidence from human brain imaging studies also indicate that cortical pathways once thought to be sensory specific can be modulated by signals from other sensory modalities.[18–22]

This more integrated view of sensory organization can be traced in part to the ground-breaking work of the perceptual psychologists James J. Gibson[23,24] and Eleanor Gibson.[25] In a sharp break from the traditional association views of perceptual development described earlier, the Gibsons recognized that the existence of different forms of sensory stimulation was not a problem for the perception of unitary events but instead provided an important basis for it. They argued that all senses should be considered as a perceptual system that interacts and works together to pick up invariant aspects of stimulation. One important type of invariant information is amodal information that is common across the senses. Amodal information is not specific to a particular sensory modality but can be conveyed redundantly across multiple senses. For example, the rhythm or tempo of a ball bouncing can be conveyed visually or acoustically and is completely redundant across the 2 senses. One can detect the same rhythm and tempo by watching the ball's motion or by listening to its impact sounds. The sight and sound of hands clapping likewise share temporal synchrony, a common tempo of action, and a common rhythm.

It is known from developmental research conducted over the past 30 years, inspired in large part by the Gibsons' innovative approach to perception, that young infants are adept perceivers of amodal information.[10,26–28] Infants readily detect the temporal aspects of stimulation, such as synchrony, rhythm, tempo, and prosody, that unite visual and acoustic stimulation from objects and events, as well as spatial co-location of objects and their sound sources and changes in intensity across the senses during the first 6 months after birth.[29,30] Such demonstrations of infants' detection of amodal information seriously question the notion that young perceivers have to learn to coordinate and somehow put together separate and distinct sources of information. By detecting higher-order amodal information common to more than one sense modality, even relatively naive perceivers can explore a unitary multimodal event in a coordinated manner. The major task of perceptual development then becomes to differentiate increasingly more specific information through detecting invariant patterns across both multimodal and unimodal sensory stimulation.[24,25,31] During perinatal development, selective attention seems to be readily biased toward stimulus properties that are common or redundant across sensory modalities.[32,33]

THE SALIENCE OF INTERSENSORY REDUNDANCY DURING EARLY DEVELOPMENT

To provide an organizing conceptual framework for defining the conditions that facilitate selective attention and perceptual learning during early development, Bahrick and Lickliter[34–36] have proposed and provided converging evidence across species (human and quail), developmental periods (prenatal and postnatal), and skill domains (discrimination, learning, memory) in support of the Intersensory Redundancy Hypothesis (IRH). The IRH is a framework that describes how selective attention is allocated to different properties of objects and events in multimodal and unimodal stimulation. The IRH was derived from the application of a convergent-operations approach[27] that designs studies that can pursue parallel research questions across human and nonhuman animal subjects to identify developmental principles involved in early intersensory perception. In brief, the IRH addresses how the detection of amodal information (not specific to any one sense modality, such as rhythm, tempo, duration, and intensity) can guide selective attention and learning during early infancy and how this process is coordinated with the perception of modality-specific information (specific to the individual sensory systems, such as color or pitch). Findings from both animal-based and human-based research consistently indicate that intersensory redundancy (the same information simultaneously available and temporally synchronized across 2 or more senses) promotes attention and perceptual processing of amodal properties of stimulation at the expense of other stimulus properties, particularly when attentional resources are most limited, such as during early development.[35,36]

The IRH has proven to be a useful framework for advancing the understanding of the emergence and maintenance of several perceptual and cognitive skills observed during infancy, including the development of affect discrimination,[37] rhythm and tempo discrimination,[38] numerical discrimination,[39,40] sequence detection,[41] abstract rule learning,[42] and word comprehension and segmentation.[43,44] These studies have all shown that intersensory redundancy can facilitate earlier and better detection of amodal information available in multimodal than in unimodal stimulation.

PRENATAL INTERSENSORY STIMULATION

The prenatal environment provides the fetus a variety of tactile, vestibular, chemical, and auditory sensory information.[45–50] Although little research has directly focused on this issue, the human fetus likely experiences a great deal of integrated multimodal stimulation across the auditory, vestibular, and tactile senses in utero. For example, when the mother walks, the sounds of her footsteps can be coordinated with tactile feedback as the fetus experiences changing pressure corresponding with the temporal patterning and shifting intensity of her movements, as well as accompanying and coordinated vestibular changes. In addition, the mother's speech sounds, laughter, heart beat, or sounds of breathing may create tactile stimulation that shares the temporal patterning of the sounds as a result of changes in the musculature involved in producing the sounds.

Fetuses also engage in spontaneous motor activity of limbs and body,[51] providing themselves temporally organized cyclic stimulation. When the fetus moves in the uterus, the movement generates both proprioceptive feedback as well as temporally coordinated tactile consequences of the motion, such as changes in pressure on the skin. In addition, the mother also responds with temporally coordinated movements to externally generated sounds. For example, she may dance or exercise to music, startle to a loud noise, or engage in conversation that has a distinctive turn-taking contingent structure, all of which produce movements that have tactile and/or vestibular correlates that share intensity and temporal patterning with the sounds. Thus, the fetus likely has ample opportunity to become familiar with and detect redundant stimulation across the various senses during the late stages of prenatal development. The role of this prenatal intersensory experience in the normal development of sensory integration and organization is currently not well understood.

It is certainly the case that during prenatal and postnatal development, fetuses and infants are ongoingly exposed to self-generated and externally generated multisensory stimulation. Evidence from research with both nonhuman animals and human fetuses and infants indicates that the specific stimulation histories of the sensory systems during prenatal and early postnatal development plays a key role in the development of selective attention, as well as early perceptual and cognitive development.[27,32,35] Of course, experiential manipulations of human fetuses and neonates are necessarily limited in scope and duration, and the traditional experimental manipulations used with animal subjects, such as sensory deprivation or sensory augmentation, are generally prohibited. As a result of these necessary restrictions, animal-based research has provided most of the advances in the understanding of the emergence of intersensory organization, including the importance of the timing of sensory experience during perinatal development,[52–56] the strong intermodal linkages of the sensory modalities during perinatal development,[57–60] and the critical role of intersensory redundancy in guiding and shaping early selective attention and, in turn, perception, learning, and memory.[32,61,62]

One obvious advantage of the use of animal subjects to study sensory organization and perceptual development in the perinatal period is the ability to readily alter both the timing and amount of particular sensory experience available to the developing fetus. Animal-based research using sensory deprivation or sensory augmentation during the perinatal period have yielded a useful body of information regarding the experiential conditions necessary for the normal development of early sensory and perceptual organization in animal infants.[52,63–69] This body of research has demonstrated that patterns of sensory stimulation available during the prenatal period actively shape emerging perceptual and cognitive capabilities. More specifically, this research indicates that the specific effects that sensory experience have on early perceptual development and sensory integration depend on several interrelated factors, including (1) the timing of sensory experience, (2) the amount of sensory experience, and (3) the type of sensory experience encountered by the fetus or the newborn.[70]

STRUCTURE/FUNCTION DYNAMICS ACROSS THE SENSORY SYSTEMS

It is important to keep in mind that the various sensory systems do not start out at birth on equal footing. This is the case because the sensory systems of birds and mammals, including humans, do not become functional at the same time in prenatal development. Rather, the sensory systems become functional in a specific and invariant sequence across early development: tactile>vestibular>chemical>auditory>visual.[46,71,72] As a result, because of the timing of their onset of function, the various sensory modalities have markedly different developmental histories at the time of birth. For example, the earlier developing tactile and vestibular systems have had much more experience during the late stages of gestation than has the later developing auditory system. These temporal dynamics likely have significant consequences for the course of early postnatal perceptual development[49] and much remains to be learned about links between the order and timing of prenatal sensory experience and subsequent postnatal perceptual processing.

Turkewitz and Kenny[73] proposed that the differential timing of sensory system onset provides a context in which earlier developing sensory systems can develop without competition or interference from later developing sensory systems. One approach to examining the importance of asynchronous sensory development is to alter the time when particular sensory input would normally be present during the perinatal period. Using this approach, Lickliter[53] found that the introduction of unusually early prenatal visual experience interfered with species-typical auditory responsiveness in bobwhite quail chicks after hatching. Chicks that experienced patterned light before hatching did not exhibit a naive preference for their species-specific maternal call, a reliable phenomenon in chicks not receiving prenatal visual stimulation. Related research demonstrated that increasing the amount of tactile and vestibular stimulation availability prenatally likewise altered postnatal auditory and visual responsiveness in quail chicks.[74] Importantly, differences in the timing of augmented prenatal stimulation led to different patterns of auditory and visual responsiveness after hatching. No effect on normal visual responsiveness to maternal cues was found when exposure to tactile and vestibular stimulation coincided with the emergence of visual function, but when exposure took place after the onset of visual functioning, chicks displayed enhanced responsiveness to the same maternal visual cues. When augmented tactile and vestibular stimulation coincided with the onset of auditory function, embryos subsequently failed to learn a species-typical maternal call before hatching. However, when given exposure to the same type and amount of augmented stimulation following the onset of auditory function, embryos did successfully learn the individual maternal call.[66] These findings indicate that augmented stimulation to earlier-emerging sensory modalities can either facilitate or interfere with perceptual responsiveness in later-developing modalities, depending on when the modified prenatal stimulation takes place.

CHANGES IN SENSORY ORGANIZATION ASSOCIATED WITH CHANGES IN SENSORY EXPERIENCE

The limited sensory capacities of the embryo and fetus (as a result of the sequential onset of sensory system function prenatally) and the constrained and buffered developmental context of the uterus combine to effectively limit and regulate the relative amount, type, and timing of sensory stimulation available during the prenatal period. These limited and regulated patterns of sensory stimulation associated with prenatal development are profoundly disrupted by preterm birth. Infants born weeks or even months before term receive dramatically altered amounts, types, and timing of sensory stimulation when compared with full-term infants. These include significant modifications in normal patterns of somesthetic, vestibular, proprioceptive, olfactory, auditory, and visual stimulation.[70] For example, the preterm infant in the neonatal intensive care unit (NICU) receives decreased amounts of some types of sensory stimulation normally available in utero (tactile and vestibular stimulation from maternal motion) and substantially increased amounts of other types of stimulation not present in the interuterine environment (unfiltered auditory stimulation and patterned visual stimulation). The perceptual and cognitive consequences of these alterations in light, sound, and movement are currently not well understood, but studies have suggested that the atypical sensory environment provided the high risk preterm infants in the NICU can have enduring effects on the developing premature brain.[75,76]

Although little is known at present about how infants integrate multisensory information at the neural level,[77,78] research from animal-based research suggests that modifications of normal patterns of perinatal sensory experience can have significant effects on early brain growth and development. For example, Markham and colleagues[79] presented augmented amounts of auditory stimulation to bobwhite quail embryos during early, middle, or late prenatal development and then tested postnatal responsiveness to species-typical auditory and visual cues. Embryos receiving auditory stimulation during middle or late stages of prenatal development showed altered postnatal visual responsiveness when compared with controls. Prenatally stimulated birds also showed a greater number of cells per unit volume of brain tissue in deep optic tectum, a midbrain region implicated in multisensory function. These results indicate that modified sensory experience delivered during prenatal development can have effects on postnatal multimodal perception as well as on the developmental trajectory of brain growth and development. These effects were temporally strained, in that when the sensory modification occurred mattered.

Working at the neurophysiologic level of analysis, Wallace and Stein[69] provided a striking example of the neural consequences of being reared in a modified species-atypical environment. In this study, domestic cats were raised from birth to adulthood in highly controlled sensory environments that allowed the systematic manipulation of the temporal and spatial features of audiovisual experience. Cats reared in this modified sensory environment, in which visual and auditory stimuli were paired to be temporally synchronous, but originated from different locations (spatially disparate), showed significant changes in the neural activity evoked by multisensory events. In particular, neurons located in superior colliculus developed a form of multisensory integration in which spatially disparate audiovisual stimuli were integrated in the same way that neurons in normally reared cats integrate audiovisual stimuli from the same location. Similarly, King and Carlile[80] found that ferrets deprived of visual experience during early development show abnormal topography and precision of spatial tuning of individual neurons in their superior colliculus, resulting in the misalignment of their auditory and visual spatial maps.

Similar results have also been reported in human-based research. Le Grand and colleagues[81] compared face processing in normal individuals with those for whom visual input had been restricted to one hemisphere from birth until 2 to 6 months of age because of congenital cataracts. The investigators found that even after more than 9 years of recovery, early deprivation of visual input to the right hemisphere severely impaired conural face processing, whereas early deprivation to the left hemisphere did not. These results are particularly striking in that when visual stimulation was delayed by as little as 2 months, permanent deficits were observed.

Sensory deprivation or augmentation in one sensory modality can also have effects on the development of the other senses.[52,53,82] Studies of deaf and blind humans have provided a wealth of evidence of increased capabilities and compensatory expansion in their remaining modalities.[83] For example, individuals who become blind early in life can process sounds faster, localize sounds more accurately, and have sharper auditory spatial tuning than sighted individuals.[84,85] Deafness likewise leads to a change in the spatial distribution of visual attention, with an enhancement of visual attention toward the peripheral visual field.[86,87] Putzar and colleagues[88,89] recently documented that human adults deprived of visual experience during the first 5 to 24 months after birth as a result of congenital cataracts show reduced audiovisual interactions as adults. Individuals who received early visual deprivation were impaired in both face recognition and in integrating auditory and visual speech signals when compared with controls. In this study, multisensory capacities had not fully recovered in adulthood, even after at least 14 years of visual experience after cataract removal.

Taken together, these animal- and human-based studies of sensory augmentation and sensory deprivation suggest that neural plasticity in early development is considerable. This plasticity is developmentally determined and allows neural systems to adjust to perturbations in the internal or external environment. It seems that neural plasticity allows sensory experience during early development to leave lasting structural and functional changes in the brain that can influence the nature and course of intersensory interactions. For concerns with care of the preterm infant, plastic changes across brain systems and related behavior vary as a function of the timing and nature of changes in experience.[83]

IMPLICATIONS FOR CARE OF THE HIGH-RISK PRETERM INFANT

Growing appreciation of the plasticity and experience-dependent nature of early sensory organization underscores the complexity of the challenge of identifying optimal care and management of the high-risk preterm infant. What will be effective or optimal for a preterm infant is a function of many interrelated factors, including at the very least their sensory and perceptual capacities, the maturity and integrity of their nervous system, and the particular characteristics of the sensory stimulation provided or denied.

In light of the remarkable plasticity of sensory organization during early development, the significant modifications of sensory experience that come with preterm birth are likely to have a range of effects on the normal course of the development of sensory organization. That being said, investigators are a long way from understanding the particulars. Given that auditory experience is typically available prenatally and that visual experience is not normally available until after birth, is there some necessary period or level of auditory experience in the period before birth for the emergence of normal patterns of postnatal perception? Does the unusually early visual experience associated with preterm birth and the resulting dramatic increase in the intensity and amount of auditory and visual stimulation interfere with normal auditory or visual development? What kinds of sensory stimulation is the fetus, preterm infant, and full-term infant particularly sensitive to? These important questions remain mostly unanswered at present. Further, little conclusive evidence is currently available about when, how much, and what type of sensory stimulation regimes are best suited to promote optimal outcomes during the various developmental stages associated with the perinatal period.

As briefly reviewed earlier, it is known that the sensory systems are strongly linked in the fetus and the neonate, such that alterations in sensory stimulation presented to one sense can result in changes in responsiveness not only in that modality but also in other sensory systems as well. It is also known that detection of amodal stimulus properties, such as synchrony, intensity, tempo, and rhythm, is promoted by redundancy across sensory modalities and is involved in the emergence of normal patterns of perceptual organization. Young infants must learn to selectively attend to relevant information, screen out irrelevant information, and efficiently detect which patterns of sensory stimulation constitute unitary multimodal events (eg, the face and voice of a person speaking) and which patterns are unrelated. These emerging skills are facilitated by intersensory processing and the detection of redundant amodal information, including temporal synchrony, rhythm, tempo, and intensity.[36]

The nature of delivery of the stimuli that preterm infants are exposed to in the NICU may, however, reduce the amount or availability of intersensory redundancy and, in turn, be detrimental to the development of early sensory integration.[70,90] For example, conditions in the NICU often do not allow preterm infants to experience stimulation in one modality concurrent with stimulation in other sensory modalities. In the full-term newborn, auditory stimulation typically results in an orienting response, a turning of the eyes in the direction of the sound source. This allows the infant to perceive the auditory and visual characteristics of the object or event from which the sound originates. In the NICU, sound sources are often not visible to the infant, even if the infant is able to turn toward them. Sounds (such as respiratory and monitoring equipment) typically occur independent of stimulation to other sensory modalities and provide little if any opportunity for the infant to match a particular sound with its visual and tactile referents. The short-term and possible long-term consequences of this reduced opportunity for intersensory redundancy on the preterm infant's emerging patterns of selective attention, perceptual processing, and learning are at present unknown. Social events provide high amounts of sensory redundancy relative to most nonsocial events. Parents and other caretakers can provide social stimulation to the high-risk infant that contains a great deal of amodal redundancy across tactile, auditory, and visual sensory systems. For example, audiovisual speech is rich with intersensory redundancy uniting the tempo, rhythm, and intensity shifts across faces and voices. This multimodal and redundant stimulation fosters the emergence of social orienting in early development by attracting and maintaining selective attention to faces, voices, and audiovisual speech. This can in turn promote early social development, as well as related perceptual and cognitive development.

Recent research has indicated that multisensory integration skills are associated with the development of intellectual abilities in school-aged children.[91] In particular, children with enhanced multisensory integration in quiet and noisy conditions were more likely to score above average on the Wechsler Intelligence Scale for Children. This finding underscores the need for additional studies on the availability and effective use of intersensory experiences in the NICU environment. Shifting the focus of study from whether experience contributes to intersensory development to how particular experiences at particular times influence intersensory development can enhance progress in the design of care and intervention programs for infants born at different levels of prematurity. There still lies a long way to achieve this challenging goal, and more studies that include the biology, behavior, and environment of the preterm in the experimental design are needed. Theoretical frameworks and statistical and modeling tools that effectively address the interactive effects that occur across these levels of analysis are also needed.

SUMMARY

The last 2 decades have seen a dramatic increase in research activity on multisensory integration. Information drawn from a range of organisms, including humans, has advanced the knowledge of developmental dynamics involved in early sensory organization. Data indicate that the sensory systems do not develop in isolation. Rather, these systems develop and function in concert with other sensory systems, even during the prenatal period. Converging evidence from behavioral, neurophysiologic, and neuroimaging studies are providing a new way of thinking about the development of sensory organization and multisensory perception. This new framework recognizes that the young brain is able to integrate input from various sensory systems to maximize the information available for perception and action. This framework also highlights the remarkable degree of neural plasticity present during early development, raising important and challenging questions about how to best manage the sensory environment of the preterm infant. More than a decade of research suggests that the nature of the delivery of sensory experience that preterm infants receive in the

NICU can overstimulate later developing sensory systems (ie, auditory and visual) and understimulate earlier developing systems (ie, tactile and vestibular), while also reducing the amount and availability of intersensory redundancy, which has been shown to be important to early selective attention, multisensory processing, and emergence of normal patterns of early perceptual organization. Investigators are still a long way from understanding the specific pathways and processes by which this unique sensory ecology of the NICU influences perceptual, behavioral, and cognitive development, and additional research is required to make informed decisions regarding how to best support the optimal development of the preterm infant.

REFERENCES

1. Birch HG, Lefford A. Intersensory development in children. Monogr Soc Res Child Dev 1963;28:3–48.
2. Friedes D. Human information processing and sensory modality: cross-modal functions, information complexity, memory, and deficit. Psychol Bull 1974;81: 284–310.
3. Piaget J. The origins of intelligence in children. New York: International Universities Press; 1952.
4. Piaget J. The construction of reality in the child. New York: Basic Books; 1954.
5. Piaget J, Inhelder B. The child's conception of space. London: Routledge; 1967.
6. Calvert G, Spence C, Stein B. The handbook of multisensory processes. Cambridge (MA): MIT Press; 2004.
7. Spelke E. Infants' intermodal perception of events. Cogn Psychol 1976;8:553–60.
8. Mendelson M, Haith M. The relation between audition and vision in the human newborn. Monogr Soc Res Child Dev 1976;41:1–72.
9. Bahrick LE, Walker AS, Neisser U. Selective looking by infants. Cogn Psychol 1981;13:377–90.
10. Lewkowicz DJ. The development of intersensory temporal perception: an epigenetic systems/limitations view. Psychol Bull 2000;126:281–308.
11. Lewkowicz DJ. Infant perception of audio-visual speech synchrony. Dev Psychol 2010;46:66–77.
12. Ernst MO, Bulthoff HH. Merging the senses into a robust percept. Trends Cogn Sci 2004;8:162–9.
13. Ghazanfar A, Schroeder C. Is neocortex essentially multisensory? Trends Cogn Sci 2006;10:278–85.
14. Gori M, Mazzilli G, Sandini G, et al. Cross-sensory facilitation reveals neural interactions between visual and tactile motion in humans. Front Psychol 2011; 2:1–9.
15. Koelewijn T, Bronkhorst A, Theeuwes J. Attention and the multiple stages of multisensory integration: a review of audiovisual studies. Acta Psychol 2010;134(3): 372–84.
16. Stein B, Meredith A. The merging of the senses. Cambridge (MA): MIT Press; 1993.
17. Zahar Y, Reches A, Gutfreund Y. Multisensory enhancement in the optic tectum of the barn owl: spike count and spike timing. J Neurophysiol 2009;101:2380–94.
18. Bushara KO, Grafman J, Hallet M. Neural correlates of auditory-visual stimulus onset asynchrony detection. J Neurosci 2001;21:300–4.
19. Driver J, Noesselt T. Multisensory interplay reveals crossmodal influences on sensory-specific brain regions, neural responses, and judgements. Neuron 2008;57:11–23.

20. Giard MH, Peronnet F. Auditory-visual integration during multimodal object recognition in humans: a behavioral and electrophysiological study. J Cogn Neurosci 1999;11:473–90.
21. Calvert GA. Crossmodal processing in the human brain: insights from functional neuroimaging studies. Cereb Cortex 2001;11:1110–23.
22. Macaluso E, Frith CD, Driver J. Modulation of human visual cortex by crossmodal spatial attention. Science 2000;289:1206–8.
23. Gibson JJ. The senses considered as perceptual systems. Boston: Houghton Mifflin; 1966.
24. Gibson JJ. The ecological approach to visual perception. Boston: Houghton Mifflin; 1979.
25. Gibson EJ. Principles of perceptual learning and development. New York: Oxford University Press; 1969.
26. Bahrick LE, Pickens J. Amodal relations: the basis for intermodal perception and learning in infancy. In: Lewkowicz DJ, Lickliter R, editors. The development of intersensory perception: comparative perspectives. Hillsdale (NJ): Erlbaum; 1994. p. 205–33.
27. Lickliter R, Bahrick LE. The development of infant intersensory perception: advantages of a comparative convergent-operations approach. Psychol Bull 2000;126:260–80.
28. Walker-Andrews AS. Infants' perception of expressive behaviors: differentiation of multimodal information. Psychol Bull 1997;121:437–56.
29. Lewkowicz DJ, Lickliter R. The development of intersensory perception: comparative perspectives. Hillsdale (NJ): Erlbaum; 1994.
30. Rose S, Ruff H. Cross modal abilities in human infants. In: Osofsky J, editor. Handbook of infant development. New York: Wiley; 1987. p. 318–62.
31. Stoffregen TA, Bardy BG. On specification and the senses. Behav Brain Sci 2001; 24:195–261.
32. Lickliter R, Bahrick LE, Honeycutt H. Intersensory redundancy facilitates prenatal perceptual learning in bobwhite quail embryos. Dev Psychol 2002;38:15–23.
33. Kraebel KS, Spear NE. Infant rats are more likely than adolescents to orient differentially to amodal features of single-element and compound stimuli. Dev Psychobiol 2000;36:49–66.
34. Bahrick LE, Lickliter R. Intersensory redundancy guides attentional selectivity and perceptual learning in infancy. Dev Psychol 2000;36:190–201.
35. Bahrick LE, Lickliter R. Intersensory redundancy guides early perceptual and cognitive development. Adv Child Dev Behav 2002;30:153–87.
36. Bahrick LE, Lickliter R. The role of intersensory redundancy in early perceptual, cognitive, and social development. In: Bremner A, Lewkowicz DJ, Spence C, editors. Multisensory development. New York: Oxford University Press; in press.
37. Flom R, Bahrick LE. The development of infant discrimination of affect in multimodal and unimodal stimulation: the role of intersensory redundancy. Dev Psychol 2007;43:238–52.
38. Bahrick LE, Lickliter R, Castellanos I, et al. Intersensory redundancy and tempo discrimination in infancy: the roles of task difficulty and expertise. Dev Sci 2010; 13:731–7.
39. Farzin F, Charles E, Rivara S. Development of multimodal processing in infancy. Infancy 2009;14:563–78.
40. Jordon KE, Suanda SH, Brannon EM. Intersensory redundancy accelerates preverbal numerical competence. Cognition 2008;108:210–21.
41. Lewkowicz DJ. Perception of serial order in infants. Dev Sci 2004;7:175–84.

42. Frank MC, Slemmer J, Marcus G, et al. Information from multiple modalities helps 5-month-olds learn abstract rules. Dev Sci 2009;12:504–9.
43. Gogate L, Bahrick LE. Intersensory redundancy and seven-month-old infants' memory for arbitrary syllable-object relations. Infancy 2001;2:219–31.
44. Hollich G, Newman RS, Jusczyk PW. Infants' use of synchronized visual information to separate streams of speech. Child Dev 2005;76:598–613.
45. DeCasper AJ, Fifer WP. Of human bonding: newborns prefer their mothers' voices. Science 1980;208:1174–6.
46. Gottlieb G. Ontogenesis of sensory function in birds and mammals. In: Tobach E, Aronson L, Shaw E, editors. The biopsychology of development. New York: Academic Press; 1971. p. 67–128.
47. Hepper PG, Scott D, Shahidullah S. Newborn and fetal response to maternal voice. J Reprod Infant Psychol 1993;11:147–53.
48. Lickliter R. Embryonic sensory experience and intersensory development in precocial birds. In: Lecanuet JP, Fifer WP, Krasnegor N, et al, editors. Fetal development: a psychobiological perspective. Hillsdale (NJ): Erlbaum; 1995. p. 281–94.
49. Lickliter R. Prenatal sensory ecology and experience: implications for perceptual and behavioral development in precocial birds. Adv Stud Behav 2005;35:235–74.
50. Smotherman W, Robinson SR. Environmental determinants of behaviour in the rat fetus. Anim Behav 1986;34:1859–73.
51. Lecanuet JP, Fifer WP, Krasnegor N, et al, editors. Oscillation and chaos in fetal motor activity. In: Fetal development: a psychobiological perspective. Hillsdale (NJ): Erlbaum; 1995. p. 169–89.
52. Kenny P, Turkewitz G. Effects of unusually early visual stimulation on the development of homing behavior in the rat pup. Dev Psychobiol 1986;19:57–66.
53. Lickliter R. Premature visual experience accelerates intersensory functioning in bobwhite quail neonates. Dev Psychobiol 1990;23:15–27.
54. Lickliter R. Timing and the development of perinatal perceptual organization. In: Turkewitz G, Devenny DA, editors. Developmental time and timing. Hillsdale (NJ): Erlbaum; 1993. p. 105–23.
55. Sleigh MJ, Lickliter R. Timing of the presentation of prenatal auditory stimulation affects postnatal perceptual responsiveness in bobwhite quail chicks. J Comp Psychol 1998;112:153–60.
56. Spear NE, McKinzie DL. Intersensory integration in the infant rat. In: Lewkowicz DJ, Lickliter R, editors. The development of intersensory perception: comparative perspectives. Hillsdale (NJ): Erlbaum; 1994. p. 133–61.
57. Gottlieb G, Tomlinson WT, Radell P. Developmental intersensory interference: premature visual experience suppresses auditory learning in ducklings. Infant Behav Dev 1989;12:1–12.
58. Lickliter R, Lewkowitz DJ. Intersensory experience and early perceptual development: attenuated prenatal sensory stimulation affects postnatal auditory and visual responsiveness in bobwhite quail chicks. Dev Psychol 1995; 31:609–18.
59. Lickliter R, Stoumbos J. Enhanced prenatal auditory experience facilitates postnatal visual responsiveness in bobwhite quail chicks. J Comp Psychol 1991;105: 89–94.
60. Radell P, Gottlieb G. Developmental intersensory interference: augmented prenatal sensory experience interferes with auditory learning in duck embryos. Dev Psychol 1992;28:795–803.
61. Lickliter R, Bahrick LE, Honeycutt H. Intersensory redundancy enhances memory in bobwhite quail embryos. Infancy 2004;5:253–69.

62. Lickliter R, Bahrick LE, Markham RG. Intersensory redundancy educates selective attention in bobwhite quail embryos. Dev Sci 2006;9(6):605–16.

63. Foreman N, Altaha M. The development of exploration and spontaneous alteration in hooded rat pups: effects of unusually early eyelid opening. Dev Psychobiol 1991;24:521–37.

64. Gottlieb G. Conceptions of prenatal development: behavioral embryology. Psychol Rev 1976;83:215–34.

65. Gottlieb G. Synthesizing nature-nurture: prenatal origins of instinctive behavior. Mahwah (NJ): Erlbaum; 1997.

66. Honeycutt H, Lickliter R. The influence of prenatal tactile and vestibular stimulation on auditory and visual responsiveness in bobwhite quail: a matter of timing. Dev Psychobiol 2003;43(2):71–81.

67. Knudsen EI, Brainard MS. Creating a unified representation of visual and auditory space in the brain. Annu Rev Neurosci 1995;18:19–43.

68. Tees R, Symons LA. Intersensory coordination and the effects of early sensory deprivation. Dev Psychobiol 1987;20:497–508.

69. Wallace MT, Stein BE. Early experience determines how the senses will interact. J Neurophysiol 2007;97:921–6.

70. Lickliter R. The role of sensory stimulation in perinatal development: insights from comparative research for care of the high-risk infant. J Dev Behav Pediatr 2000; 21:437–47.

71. Alberts J. Sensory-perceptual development in the Norway rat: a view toward comparative studies. In: Kail R, Spear N, editors. Comparative perspectives on memory development. Hillsdale (NJ): Erlbaum; 1984. p. 65–101.

72. Bradley RM, Mistretta CM. Fetal sensory receptors. Physiol Rev 1975;55:352–82.

73. Turkewitz G, Kenny P. The role of developmental limitation of sensory input on sensory/perceptual organization. J Dev Behav Pediatr 1985;6:302–6.

74. Carlsen RM, Lickliter R. Augmented prenatal tactile and vestibular stimulation alters postnatal auditory and visual responsiveness in bobwhite quail chicks. Dev Psychobiol 1999;35(3):215–25.

75. Als H, Gilkerson L, Duffy F, et al. A three-center, randomized, controlled trial of individualized developmental care for very low birth weight preterm infants: medical, neurodevelopmental, parenting, and caregiving effects. J Dev Behav Pediatr 2003;24:399–408.

76. Gressens P, Rogido M, Paindaveine B, et al. The impact of the neonatal intensive care practices on the developing brain. J Pediatr 2002;140:646–53.

77. Hyde DC, Jones BL, Porter CL, et al. Visual stimulation enhances auditory processing in 3-month-old infants and adults. Dev Psychobiol 2010;52:181–9.

78. Hyde DC, Jones BL, Flom R, et al. Neural signatures of face-voice synchrony in 5-month-old infants. Dev Psychobiol 2011;53:359–70.

79. Markham R, Shimizu T, Lickliter R. Extrinsic embryonic sensory stimulation alters multimodal behavior and cellular activation. Dev Neurobiol 2008;68:1463–73.

80. King AJ, Carlile S. Changes induced in the representation of auditory space in the superior colliculus by rearing ferrets with binocular eyelid suture. Exp Brain Res 1993;94:444–55.

81. Le Grand R, Mondloch CJ, Maurer D, et al. Expert face processing requires visual input to the right hemisphere during infancy. Nat Neurosci 2003;6:1108–12.

82. Lickliter R. Prenatal visual experience alters postnatal sensory dominance hierarchy in bobwhite quail chicks. Infant Behav Dev 1994;17:185–93.

83. Bavelier D, Neville HJ. Cross-modal plasticity: where and how? Nat Rev Neurosci 2004;3:443–52.

84. Lessard N, Pare M, Leore F, et al. Early-blind human subjects localize sound sources better than sighted subjects. Nature 1998;395:278–80.
85. Roder B, Teder-Salejarvi W, Sterr A, et al. Improved auditory spatial tuning in blind humans. Nature 1999;400:162–6.
86. Neville HJ, Lawson DS. Attention to central and peripheral visual space in a movement detection task: an event related potential and behavioral study. II. Congenitially deaf adults. Brain Res 1987;405:268–83.
87. Stivalet P, Moreno Y, Richard J, et al. Differences in visual search tasks between congenitally deaf and normally hearing adults. Brain Res Cogn Brain Res 1998;6: 227–32.
88. Putzar L, Goerendt I, Lange K, et al. Early visual deprivation impairs multisensory interactions in humans. Nat Neurosci 2007;10:1243–5.
89. Putzar L, Hotting K, Roder B. Early visual deprivation affects the development of face recognition and of audio-visual speech perception. Restor Neurol Neurosci 2010;28:251–7.
90. Lawson K, Daum C, Turkewitz G. Environmental characteristics of a neonatal intensive care unit. Child Dev 1977;48:1633–9.
91. Barutchu A, Crewther SG, Pifer J, et al. The relationship between multisensory integration and IQ in children. Dev Psychol 2011;47:877–85.

Motor System Development of the Preterm and Low Birthweight Infant

Julia B. Pitcher, PhD[a],*, Luke A. Schneider, PhD[a],
John L. Drysdale, BAppSc(Phty) Hons[a], Michael C. Ridding, PhD[a],
Julie A. Owens, PhD[b]

KEYWORDS

- Motor system development • Preterm infant
- Low birthweight infant

Impaired motor and cognitive development remain the 2 major adverse outcomes of preterm birth, despite advances in neonatal care.[1] Up to 50% of preterm children without cerebral palsy have motor difficulties and show adverse neurologic signs at school age that, although often subtle, substantially affect their motor and cognitive development, educational achievement, and social adjustment.[2–7] These developmental difficulties are not confined to the very preterm. There is emerging evidence that late preterm children (ie, those born between 33 and 36 completed weeks' gestational age [GA]) also experience significant motor, cognitive, and behavioral difficulties at school age. The importance of this neglected area of child health was recently highlighted in several editorials in the *Journal of Pediatrics*, in which the issue of the health of the late preterm child was identified as a "new disease."[8–10] This motor and cognitive dysfunction of prematurity often co-occurs, suggesting a similar underlying pathology. New evidence in the basic science literature indicates that the motor areas of the brain also contribute to cognitive processes, including speech perception and

This work was supported by research grants from the Australian National Health and Medical Research Council (299087 and 565344), the M.S. McLeod Trust, the Women's and Children's Hospital Research Foundation and the South Australian Channel 7 Children's Research Foundation.

The authors have nothing to disclose.

[a] Neuromotor Plasticity and Development, DX 650-517 Robinson Institute, Discipline of Obstetrics and Gynaecology, School of Paediatrics and Reproductive Health, University of Adelaide, Adelaide, Australia

[b] Research Centre for the Early Origins of Health and Disease, DX 650-521 Robinson Institute, Discipline of Obstetrics and Gynaecology, School of Paediatrics and Reproductive Health, University of Adelaide, Adelaide, Australia

* Corresponding author.

E-mail address: julia.pitcher@adelaide.edu.au

learning.[11–13] This finding casts new light on the large body of work regarding the influence of very preterm birth on age-appropriate development of both motor and cognitive functions and similar findings emerging for the late preterm. However, little is known of the changes in the physiology of the neural pathways that underlies any developmental delay or dysfunction in these domains. Even the neurophysiology underpinning motor function in neurologically healthy term-born children has been little characterized. These gaps have hindered development of novel and more effective therapies and diagnostic approaches and highlight new opportunities.

In this article some of the most recent findings regarding altered motor development in children born preterm are reviewed, particularly in those children with no apparent brain lesion. The possible relationship to effects of preterm birth on cognitive function is touched on. The role of neuroplasticity in both exacerbating and improving these outcomes postnatally is explored. Because many preterm children also experience either intrauterine growth restriction (IUGR) or are born small for gestational age (SGA), some of the evidence for differential effects of shortened gestation versus suboptimal fetal growth on neurodevelopment is explored. Hypothetical scenarios are posed as to how some early developmental care practices might both help and hinder long-term outcomes for these children, for future study. Although some of the underlying physiology of some of these brain conditions associated with preterm birth is touched on, it is beyond the scope of this review to include the specific mechanisms of preterm brain injury, and readers are referred elsewhere for this.[14–16]

BRAIN DEVELOPMENT, CORTICAL FOLDING, AND CONNECTIVITY IN THE PRETERM BRAIN

Preterm birth between 20 and 37 weeks' GA corresponds to a time of rapid cortical growth, particularly in the motor and sensorimotor areas. The premature transition from the intrauterine to the extrauterine environment alters the trajectory and temporal characteristics of brain development, and the earlier the birth, the greater the perturbation from normal growth trajectories.[17] Even in the absence of focal brain lesions, many preterm children have reduced regional brain volumes and compromised development of both white and gray matter.[18–20] Critically, these abnormalities remain in late adolescence, and include major motor control areas, such as the sensorimotor, premotor, and primary motor cortices (ie, the corticospinal system), the basal ganglia and cerebellum, and the corpus callosum, the main pathway connecting the 2 brain hemispheres.[18–21] There is increasing evidence that it is the interruption to cortical development, in particular, that is likely to underlie many of the cognitive and the more subtle motor sequelae, which commonly manifest in preterm children.[22–24] Preterm infants often have reduced cortical folding (ie, gyrification) at term-equivalent age compared with their term-born peers, even in the absence of focal lesions.[17] Taken together, these structural and functional findings imply that preterm birth disrupts the normal development of functional connectivity within and between cortical regions.

Recently, functional connectivity magnetic resonance imaging (fcMRI) has been used to examine functional connectivity in resting state neural networks in the brains of preterm children.[25–27] Resting state networks refer to regions of the brain that are known to be structurally connected and show synchronized activation during specific task performance; fcMRI studies examine the neuronal activity in these networks in the resting state (ie, in the absence of task performance).[27] In adults, this method has been used to identify networks including those contributing to motor function, sensory function, language, auditory processing, and visual processing[26] (reviewed in Ref.[27]). Compared with their term-born peers, fcMRI at term-equivalent age in preterm infants has shown that these networks, including motor networks, show aberrant connectivity and are less mature, particularly the thalamocortical networks.[26] It has been proposed that some of this altered connectivity, at least later in childhood, may be compensatory and benefit from the capacity of the developing brain for neuroplastic reorganization.[28] However, the significant incidence of subtle motor and cognitive dysfunction in apparently healthy preterm children, born at a range of GAs, argues against this proposition, although studies are lacking.

The mechanisms underlying the development of aberrant functional connectivity remain unknown, although white matter damage directly disrupts corticocortical and corticothalamic connections, and gray matter damage alters the connection targets.[26] However, Smyser and colleagues[26] have suggested that an effect of the sensory experience of the preterm infant (eg, in the neonatal intensive care unit [NICU]) on functional connectivity development cannot be discounted. What also remains unknown is if and how it might be possible to therapeutically improve suboptimal brain connectivity in preterm children.

VULNERABILITY OF MOTOR NEUROPHYSIOLOGY IN THE PRETERM NEONATE

The development and performance of skilled movements of the arms, fingers, legs, and other extremities relies principally on the healthy development of the corticospinal system, the main descending pathway via which the motor cortex controls voluntary movement.[29–31] Given the multiple brain regions from which its neurons arise, it is not surprising that the corticospinal system is so susceptible to brain damage in the prenatal and neonatal periods.[32] Lesions occurring during these periods are associated with impairment in learning and performing skilled movements, and abnormal spinal reflex control associated with, for example, spasticity.[33] The pattern of brain injury seems highly dependent on GA. Cerebral white matter injuries are most common and severe in infants born between 24 and 32 weeks' GA, and predominantly include damage to premyelinating oligodendrocytes, marked microgliosis, and hypomyelination.[34] The late preterm period from around 33 to 40 weeks' GA is characterized by a rapid and voluminous growth and development of the gray matter, and vulnerability to hypoxic-ischemic injury to the cerebral cortex.[14,35] Vulnerability of the gray matter depends on the timing of the injury because different gray matter regions mature at different times. Billiards and colleagues[14] found that at mid-gestation brainstem damage predominates, followed by injury to the deep gray nuclei and the cerebral cortex at term. However, there is also a 5-fold increase in white matter volume during this period and, although the incidence is lower than in the early preterm, the late preterm brain remains vulnerable to periventricular leukomalacia.[35] In term-born neonates, most brain injuries are sequelae from hypoxic-ischemic insults. Damage often involves the white and gray matter, particularly of the cerebral cortex and hippocampus, but the extent depends on the duration and severity of the insult. Despite more than a century of research, we still do not fully understand how the brain motor areas and spinal motoneurons produce and control movements, nor the extent of and mechanisms underlying compensatory neuroplasticity when motor pathways are damaged during development or later in life.[31,36]

Recent evidence from three-dimensional (3D) tractography shows that, in normally developing humans, the corticospinal tract undergoes a protracted maturation, starting before birth and reaching at least into adolescence.[37] Although this observation implies that it is vulnerable to developmental injury for longer, it also suggests that the period during which the tract may also be receptive to ameliorative neurodevelopmental interventions may extend well past infancy and early childhood under some circumstances.

TRANSCRANIAL MAGNETIC STIMULATION STUDIES OF CORTICOSPINAL AND MOTOR CORTEX DEVELOPMENT IN PRETERM INFANTS AND CHILDREN

Transcranial magnetic stimulation (TMS) is a noninvasive, painless technique that allows stimulation of the conscious human brain through the scalp and skull. When applied over the motor cortex region at sufficient intensity, TMS activates corticospinal output neurons and results in a small contraction in, for example, the hand muscles on the opposite (ie, contralateral) side of the body. This twitch in the muscle, called the motor-evoked potential (MEP), can be measured using surface electrodes on the skin overlying the muscle. The size and latency of the MEP reflect the excitability of neurons and impulse conduction characteristics of the motor cortex, corticospinal tract, and spinal motor centers. The advent of TMS has allowed examination of the development of the motor system in humans of all ages.

The Motor Threshold

The motor threshold is the lowest intensity at which TMS of the motor cortex results in an MEP in a muscle. Diffusion-weighted imaging has shown that, in adults aged 26 to 55 years, both the resting and active motor thresholds correlate strongly with the maturation, myelination, and structural integrity of the primary motor cortex and premotor cortex white matter; lower motor thresholds correlate negatively with regional fractional anisotropy.[38] This finding has significant functional implications, because greater regional white matter fractional anisotropy is associated with increased proficiency in motor skills in children, adolescents, and adults[34,39] and suggests that the motor threshold to TMS may be a sensitive measure of motor region white matter integrity for a range of age groups. Bengtsson and colleagues' study[39] also highlights an important property of the maturing corticospinal tract and motor region white matter: white matter integrity is susceptible to activity-dependent plasticity, particularly during childhood, and practicing motor skills during this period can improve development of white matter integrity.

Nerve Conduction Velocity

Koh and Eyre[40] used TMS to describe maturation of corticospinal conduction velocity in 142 individuals ranging from preterm neonates (33 weeks' GA) to 50-year-old adults. Some of the infants were as young as 5 days old when assessed, but MEPs (recorded from biceps brachii in infants and an intrinsic hand muscle in older children and adults) could be evoked in every individual. In all children less than 8 years of age background voluntary muscle contraction was required to evoke an MEP. Between 8 and 11 years of age, the motor threshold and probability of evoking an MEP in the relaxed muscle progressively increased. Conduction velocity increased from around 10.5 meters per second (ms^{-1}) at 33 weeks to adult values of 79 ms^{-1} at 11 years. Peripheral motor nerve conduction velocity reaches adult levels by 3 years of age,[41] whereas central sensory afferent conduction is more prolonged, reaching adult values at around 8 years.[42] Koh and Eyre showed that maturation of the central motor pathways is significantly more protracted than the peripheral pathways.

A subsequent TMS study of 223 preterm and term-born neonates (26–41 weeks' GA at birth) showed that even in preterm babies, direct monosynaptic corticomotoneuronal projections are already present, and that these precede the development of the first appearance of motor skills, with acquisition of relatively independent finger movements occurring by at least 12 months.[29] However, infants show reaching and grasping movements well before this and it has been shown that absent or abnormal reaching behavior in preterm infants at 4 months and poor reaching movement quality at 6 months corrected age is associated with a poorer neuromotor outcome at 6 years of age.[43] Prediction of a child's motor outcomes at school age is often based on whether a child reached early life motor milestones within the appropriate age window. However, this approach is not only subjective but also often limited by frequent false-negative results. Neurophysiologic assessment of corticospinal development may therefore offer a useful adjunct in better predicting neuromotor outcomes in early infancy.

Cortical Excitability and Motor Development in Childhood

We have recently used TMS to investigate the effect of GA and fetal growth (as measured by birthweight centile[44,45]) on the motor threshold in 147 children (aged 11.9 ± 0.8 years) who were born at 28 to 41 weeks' GA.[46] The findings regarding birthweight centile are discussed in a later section. Age-appropriate motor skill development was assessed with the Movement Assessment Battery for Children (version 2).[47] None had any history of brain lesion or abnormal perinatal brain imaging. Motor threshold decreased linearly with increased GA in both left and right hemispheres, but locally weighted linear regression showed 3 distinct groups. Although motor threshold decreased progressively for each week of GA gained between 24 and 33 weeks, there was no further decrease in those children born after 33 weeks' but before 37 weeks' GA (ie, the late preterm children). There was then a sharp decline in motor threshold for every week of gestation gained from 38 to 41 weeks. White matter damage is most prevalent in children born at less than 32 weeks' GA[48] and is the most likely explanation for the association found between motor threshold and GA in children born at 24 and 33 weeks' GA. From 38 weeks' GA, corticospinal diameter begins to rapidly increase[29]; a possible explanation for our findings in the term children is that each week of late GA may be important in optimizing axonal development. We have previously found effects of GA within this period in term-born 28-year-old adults born at a range of birthweight centiles.[49] Functionally, a low motor threshold was a better predictor of good motor skill development than GA, particularly when parental factors and socioeconomic circumstances at the time of the child's birth were taken into account.[50]

These findings suggest that although preterm birth confers a risk of suboptimal corticospinal and function motor skill development (and the more preterm the birth the greater the risk), the postnatal environment plays a critical role in how that risk manifests. Although we lack direct evidence, taken together with Bengtsson and colleagues'[39] findings, our findings support the notion that not only is the motor threshold to TMS a sensitive measure of motor region white matter integrity in children born preterm, but that an advantageous postnatal environment can probably ameliorate at least some of the consequences of preterm birth on motor development. Given the protracted development of the corticospinal pathway, the temporal window of opportunity in which we can therapeutically manipulate this developmental plasticity to optimize neuromotor development in preterm children may be significantly wider than previously believed.

A ROLE FOR THE MOTOR CORTEX IN COGNITIVE DEVELOPMENT AND FUNCTION

A consistent finding is that up to 50% of noncerebral palsy children born before 33 weeks' GA have cognitive difficulties at school that are associated with concomitant motor dysfunction.[3,6,7,51,52] In addition to reduced motor cortex excitability,[50] the few studies of cognitive outcomes in late preterm children also show an increased risk of learning difficulties in this preterm group, particularly in the areas of reading and language.[53–55] Whether or not reduced motor cortex excitability directly contributes to reduced cognitive abilities in preterm children, or simply provides an overall indicator of cortical development, is unknown. However, there is increasing evidence that the brain motor areas contribute to higher cognitive processing, including speech and language perception, and not just to movement control.

There is ample evidence that areas in the left inferior frontal cortex (ie, Broca's area) and the superior temporal cortex (ie, Wernicke's area) play major roles in language processing. However, recent TMS, neuroimaging, and neuropsychological investigations have revealed that numerous other cortical areas, including the primary motor cortex and premotor areas, are involved in both the production of speech (ie, by activating muscles to produce speech sounds) and in its perception and interpretation, whether in the spoken word or read form.[56–59] TMS studies in healthy human adults have shown that the excitability of the motor cortex is increased by listening to speech sounds as well as during overt and covert reading.[56,58,59] This increased excitability, or facilitation, indicates engagement of the motor cortex by the speech listening (or reading) task and is indicated by an increase in the amplitude of the MEP evoked with TMS of the motor cortex. This increased excitability has been documented in speech muscles (ie, orofacial and tongue muscles)[59,60] as well as in hand and leg muscles,[56,58,61] and is believed to reflect the motor centers of the brain contributing to decoding the meaning of words. It is more pronounced when a greater effort is required to understand new or familiar words, short-term memory of strings of words (eg, to comprehend sentences when reading) or when listening to speech in a noisy environment.[59] TMS studies of patients with lesions affecting the inferior frontal regions of the brain have shown motor circuits contributing to comprehension of phonemes, semantic categories, and grammar.[61–63] Taken together, these findings suggest that a normally developing motor cortex contributes to auditory (ie, spoken words) and visual (reading) speech perception and language comprehension. Therefore, it is possible that the reduced motor cortex excitability seen in preterm children may have an adverse effect on motor cortical contributions to speech perception and interpretation in these children. We are currently testing this hypothesis in preterm children aged 11 to 12 years. However, the available evidence suggests that optimizing a preterm child's motor development may have subtle but significant effects on their cognitive outcomes.

IUGR IS DISTINCT FROM SHORTENED GESTATION

A significant proportion of infants born preterm are also growth restricted. An often-neglected problem inherent in the literature regarding neurologic development after preterm birth is that the effects of shortened gestation are not consistently distinguished from those of fetal growth restriction.[21,64] Suboptimal fetal growth is referred to as either IUGR, or being born SGA. IUGR and SGA are often used interchangeably, but by definition they are different conditions. SGA is defined by the World Health Organization as a birthweight less than the tenth percentile for GA, whereas IUGR is a pathologic condition in which the fetus is unable to grow to its genetically determined potential size, because of either abnormal genetic or environmental conditions that impair growth. So although all IUGR infants are SGA, not all SGA infants are IUGR.[64]

There is evidence that the effects of IUGR/SGA on motor system development are likely to be both direct and indirect. The direct effects include alterations in substrate supply that affect brain perfusion, growth, and development, whereas the indirect effects include adverse development of other systems (metabolic, endocrine, and cardiovascular) that secondarily influence neurodevelopment. Several imaging studies have shown that fetal growth restriction has specific effects on cortical and hippocampal structure and function that are different to those caused by shortened gestation.[65–68] In addition, term-born SGA individuals can have altered neuromotor development that persists into adulthood and is associated with a reduced likelihood of completing a university education, even without evidence of disability.[49,64] Failure to differentiate those brain changes caused by growth restriction from those caused by shortened gestation make determining causation, and therefore predicting neurodevelopmental outcome, difficult. The distinction is also important in neonatal and early childhood care, because growth-restricted infants who fail to undergo catch-up growth in the first 12 to 18 months of life are at particular risk of adverse motor and cognitive outcomes.[69–74] Overall, the current evidence suggests that growth restriction and prematurity have some similar but also some distinct outcomes for neurodevelopment and function in the short-term and long-term.

EFFECTS OF FETAL GROWTH RESTRICTION ON BRAIN DEVELOPMENT AND CORTICOSPINAL EXCITABILITY

There is a paucity of studies that have clearly differentiated the effects of fetal growth restriction on brain neurophysiology from those of preterm birth. Using 3D morphometric MRI techniques, Martinnusen and colleagues[67] showed that compared with term-born appropriately grown for GA controls, the right hemisphere cortical area was significantly reduced in term-born SGA adolescents, and there was a trend for reduced cortical volume. This finding is in contrast with the preterm group (mean GA 29.1 ± 2.7 weeks, ≤1500 g) who had reduced cortical volume and surface area in both hemispheres. Using TMS, we have previously shown in adults born at term (37–41 weeks' GA) but across a range of birthweight centiles that SGA/IUGR selectively reduces right hemisphere motor cortex excitability. Functionally, these excitability changes are associated with normal or even superior right-hand dexterity, but poorer than average left-hand skills. We have now confirmed the TMS findings in a pediatric population and shown that the effect is independent of GA.[50] In our study of 12-year-old children,[50] a lower birthweight centile (which is corrected for GA) was associated with a higher motor threshold, but only in the left hand (ie, the right motor cortex).

Brain sparing is a term used to refer to the maintenance of relative brain size compared with other organs by the fetus in response to chronically reduced intrauterine substrate supply (nutrients, oxygen) and includes a hemodynamic and a neuroendocrine response.[75,76] However, there are marked and impactful structural and functional consequences that are not prevented by this phenomenon, although these may be ameliorated to some extent and would have been worse otherwise. The hemodynamic response results in the redistribution of blood flow to favor the brain, and the neuroendocrine response by the brain reduces somatic growth rate. The MRI and TMS findings to date suggest that apparent brain sparing may be finer grained than previously believed, and favor sparing of the left hemisphere over the right in the growth-restricted fetus.

NEUROPLASTICITY AND NEUROMOTOR OUTCOME IN THE PRETERM CHILD

As we have discussed, preterm children have alterations in cortical development, functional connectivity, and patterns of neural activation in response to incoming stimuli. This finding suggests that their capacity for neuroplasticity is also reduced and may contribute to their common difficulties with learning and memory.[77] Neuroplasticity refers to the ability of the brain to make short-term or long-term modifications to the strength and number of its synaptic neuronal connections in response to incoming stimuli associated with activity and experience. There is extensive experimental evidence that this selective strengthening (long-term potentiation [LTP]) and weakening (long-term depression [LTD]) of synapses is the physiologic basis underlying learning and possibly memory, although the evidence for the latter is less clear. Neuroplasticity is a lifelong property of the human brain, although it is most prominent from birth until late childhood and early adolescence. Although not fully established, the most parsimonious explanation for neuroplasticity peaking during early life is that this period not only coincides with a period of rapid brain growth but also brain complexity, including the protracted generation of excessive new synapses (synaptogenesis) and the activity-dependent and experience-dependent pruning of synapses.

Most of our understanding of the mechanisms underlying neuroplasticity has come from animal studies using cell preparations and brain slices. However, the advent of TMS has led to an explosion of research into real-time induction of neuroplasticity in the cortices of awake humans. Apart from being a tool to assess the integrity of the motor pathways, different TMS systems (ie, rapid rate TMS [rTMS]) that can deliver preprogrammable trains of pulses can also be used to induce short-term cortical neuroplasticity. The strength and duration of the neuroplasticity induced by the rTMS train is reflected as changes in the excitability of the motor cortex and corticospinal motor pathway. This entity is measured as changes in the amplitude of the MEP to single-pulse stimulation of the motor cortex. Depending on the frequency and intensity characteristics of the pulse train, the neuroplasticity can either be LTP-like synaptic strengthening (ie, the MEP responses get larger) or LTD-like synaptic weakening (ie, the MEP responses get smaller) (**Fig. 1**). In general, the effect is relatively short-lived (about 60 minutes in healthy adults), but there is currently a large international research effort directed at developing different rTMS protocols for therapeutic use in a range of neuropathologic conditions and psychiatric disorders, with mixed success (reviewed in Ref.[78]). However, there is evidence from other studies combining rTMS with traditional therapies such as physiotherapy that rTMS may act by priming the brain to being more receptive to those therapies.

We have recently begun using rTMS to examine the capacity for short-term neuroplasticity induction in preterm children who are now 12 to 14 years of age, with no history of perinatal brain lesion. Our preliminary data[77] have yielded 2 key findings. First, the capacity for LTD-like motor neuroplasticity induction at this age in term-born children is significantly greater, both in strength and duration, than in adults. This finding confirms that the motor system is still highly plastic in early adolescence. Second, compared with their term-born peers, preterm children born at 28 to 36 weeks' GA have a significantly reduced capacity for and duration of this type of LTD-like neuroplasticity. There was no difference in neuroplasticity capacity when early preterm (25–32 weeks' GA) were compared with late preterm (33–36 weeks' GA). We are now extending this research to determine if preterm children have a similarly reduced capacity for LTP-like neuroplasticity. We are also trialling some simple interventions to determine if neuroplastic capacity can be increased in these children, and at what ages.

The capacity of the brain for neuroplastic change is not simply a function of synaptic number or strength. There are several physiologic factors that can modify an individual's capacity for neuroplastic reorganization. Two of particular interest in the developing brain are the stress hormone and glucocorticoid cortisol and a member of the neurotrophin family intimately involved in central and peripheral nervous system development, maturation, and maintenance: brain-derived neurotrophic factor (BDNF).[79] Both may mediate some of the critical effects of in utero and ex utero exposures of the IUGR and preterm infant as well as provide potential targets of interventions to restore neurodevelopment and function in such infants and children.

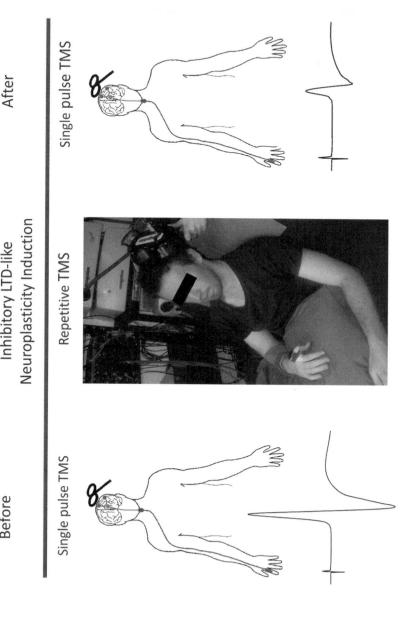

Fig. 1. LTD-like neuroplasticity induction using rTMS. Before rTMS, single-pulse TMS are applied over the hand representation in the motor cortex and the resultant MEPs recorded using surface electromyography of the contralateral index finger muscle. The middle panel shows rTMS being applied to patient's left motor cortex with the rTMS coil and the electromyography electrodes on his right index finger muscle. After LTD-like neuroplasticity induction, the amplitudes of the MEPs evoked with single-pulse TMS are depressed for up to 60 minutes in adults.

ALTERED STRESS HORMONE RESPONSIVENESS LONG-TERM MAY INFLUENCE NEUROPLASTICITY IN PRETERM CHILDREN

Intrauterine and extrauterine exposure to excess glucocorticoids is likely to be common in the preterm infant. The known common causes of preterm delivery, or factors associated with this, such as an exaggerated inflammatory state or an adverse metabolic and hormonal environment, are often characterized by increased endogenous glucocorticoids. The premature delivery of the immature neonate into the extrauterine environment can also increase endogenous glucocorticoid production and exposure. Exogenous steroids given prenatally to mature the lungs or even postnatally may add further to the extent of exposure of the preterm infant. Although beneficial for short-term survival, excess glucocorticoids in early life can also be a major initiator of programming of developmental changes that can persist.[80] This finding has been documented in humans and animal species and reviewed extensively elsewhere,[81,82] with structural, cellular, and molecular changes in the brain and in specific regions, resulting in behavioral and functional consequences. These consequences can include programming of altered responsiveness of the hypothalamopituitary-adrenal axis (HPA) itself in the short-term and long-term, with increased reactivity in later life, usually reported after prematurity[82] or IUGR.[81,83]

The interest in cortisol in terms of developmental care has largely centered on its role in the stress response in infants receiving neonatal intensive care. As outlined earlier, for the preterm neonate the ex utero environment is also highly stressful, in part because of physiologically immature organ systems being challenged by what is an inappropriate environment. Developmental care practices may modulate the extent to which this situation occurs.

Few studies have studied circadian cortisol secretion serially in either preterm or term-born neonates. The overall picture is one of considerable interindividual variation in cortisol secretion patterns and single plasma or salivary levels. For example, Bettendorf and colleagues[84] collected salivary cortisol samples from healthy term and preterm neonates every 6 hours for 3 sequential days. Mature salivary cortisol rhythms were variably established, with no clear difference with prematurity, however, glucocorticoid administration did reduce endogenous salivary cortisol in the premature neonates, a finding since confirmed by others.[85,86] Preterm birth does seem to be associated with a reduced cortisol response to critical illness and other stressors,[82,87] a pattern that persists in infancy,[88] then reverses after about 18 months and persists longer term.[81,82,89] These patterns may affect the immediate physiologic capacity of the infant to survive challenges to their immune and cardiovascular systems.

However, there is increasing recognition that the multiple sensorimotor stimuli the preterm neonate experiences ex utero can have an enduring adverse effect on their short-term and long-term neurodevelopmental outcome. There is also an increasing literature concerning possible long-term changes in stress responsiveness and neurodevelopment in infants exposed to multiple invasive painful procedures in the NICU.[89–91] Apart from procedural pain, the infant in the NICU is exposed to and must mount responses to several other potential stressors, including maternal and paternal separation, increased light and noise, the effects of acute and chronic illness, and varying combinations of too much or too little handling or tactile stimulation. Reducing the impact of these environmental stressors, particularly on short-term and long-term neurodevelopment, has formed the basis of several developmental care strategies, including the Newborn Individualised Developmental Care and Assessment Program (NIDCAP)[92] and Kangaroo Mother Care.[93]

Recently cortisol has been shown to be a powerful acute modulator of neuroplasticity in the adult human. The neuroplastic responsiveness of the brain to stimulatory input is reduced when circulating levels of cortisol are high during the normal diurnal variation that occurs.[94] Sale and colleagues[94] showed that in normal healthy adults, neuroplasticity induction is greatest in the afternoon, when diurnal cortisol is at its nadir, and lowest during the morning around the time of peak circulating cortisol. Furthermore, high neuroplastic responsiveness in the afternoon can be blocked by administering hydrocortisone.[94] These and other similar findings suggest that abnormal circulating cortisol levels, or alterations in the diurnal pattern of cortisol secretion, may limit an individual's capacity for neuroplastic reorganization and, hence, learning and memory. Measures of cortisol abundance or secretion have been related to memory recognition in preterm infants.[95]

Given the effects of cortisol on motor cortex neuroplasticity induction in adults,[94] one hypothetical mechanism by which early environment stress may influence long-term neuromotor development is by abnormally programming the HPA. In this scenario, abnormal cortisol secretion levels or circadian rhythms reduce the capacity for motor neuroplasticity and, hence, the learning and memory of motor skills. This finding is likely to be exacerbated in those preterm infants who were IUGR, because this prenatal stressor is known to program higher basal HPA axis function regardless of GA at birth.[96]

THE ROLE OF BDNF IN NEUROPLASTICITY IN THE PRETERM BRAIN

Many nervous system growth factors and neuropeptide families have roles in brain development and neuronal survival and function, but one of the most abundant and one with widespread actions throughout the brain is BDNF. BDNF is a key regulator of axonal and dendritic growth, functional connectivity,[97] peripheral nervous system myelination,[98] and neuronal survival during development. It is widely expressed in the brain, as are its receptors, particularly in the cortex, cerebellum, and hippocampus. Among an array of functions, BDNF plays a key role in neuroplasticity because it regulates synaptic structure and controls activity-dependent synaptic transmission (reviewed in Ref.[99]). In particular, BDNF signaling at synapses enhances LTP and hence learning and memory.[100] Exogenous BDNF after experimental hypoxic-ischemic injury reduces apoptotic neuronal loss and some spatial memory impairment in neonatal rats.[101–103] Limited amounts of BDNF may cross the blood-brain barrier into the brain (in the adult at least) but circulating peripheral and central nervous system levels of BDNF are closely correlated. Human in vivo studies are exploiting this relationship and using circulating BDNF as a surrogate marker of central nervous system BDNF. This close association suggests either coregulation or even transfer of BDNF between the 2 compartments in early life, when the blood-brain barrier is less mature. The diverse functions of BDNF have also led to a major focus on its therapeutic potential (ie, neuroprotection and repair) in neurologic disease and injury, notwithstanding the challenges of exogenous delivery or indirectly enhancing endogenous production.[104]

Relatively little is known of the BDNF system and brain development after preterm birth, but it seems consistent with its better-characterized actions and functions. Cord blood BDNF increases with increasing GA at birth[105] and, in the developing brain, has been shown to modulate expression of the metalloprotein reelin. Reelin is important in early cortical organization, particularly the inside-out development of the cortical layers, and is downregulated by increasing BDNF abundance as lamination is completed, synaptogenesis begins, and cortical maturity increases.[106] Hence, BDNF seems to have an important role in determining cortical maturation. Certainly, the increase in plasma BDNF levels during gestation coincides with and is reflective of increases in cortical gray matter.[105] However, BDNF is differentially expressed in various brain regions postnatally, and much of the evidence to date for a critical role of BDNF in cortical development after birth is based on events in prefrontal cortex rather than the motor cortical areas.

Circulating BDNF levels are often lower in preterm infants who go on to develop moderate to severe intraventricular hemorrhage,[105,107,108] although this might simply be reflective of their level of prematurity. Cord blood BDNF is higher in those preterm infants whose mothers had received a complete course of antenatal corticosteroids, suggesting that part of the neuroprotective effect of this treatment may be achieved via increased fetal BDNF production either in the brain or in a compartment from which BDNF can access the brain.[105,108] Possible mechanisms of action might include upregulation of fetal BDNF synthesis in response to antenatal corticosteroids or an indirect increase in fetal neuronal BDNF as a result of greater neuronal maturation after corticosteroid treatment.[105,108] By contrast, circulating BDNF levels are decreased in infants after postnatal corticosteroid treatment.[108]

The impact of transition to intrauterine life on BDNF abundance in the developing fetus and infant and the impact of prematurity on this has been characterized to a limited extent. In a study of 30 term-born (mean GA = 39.2 $\pm$ 1.4 weeks; 37–41 weeks) and 15 preterm neonates (mean GA = 29.4 $\pm$ 1.3 weeks; 28–32 weeks), Malamitsi-Puchner and colleagues[107] defined the impact of premature delivery on the antenatal changes in maternal and fetal/neonatal blood BDNF up to 4 days after delivery. Maternal blood BDNF did not vary with preterm delivery but was higher than cord blood and neonatal BDNF overall. Preterm delivery reduced blood BDNF in the newborn and the neonate, independent of mode of delivery or gender. Compared with cord blood BDNF, circulating blood BDNF was increased 24 hours after birth and, although this was maintained in term infants, it then decreased in the preterm. The former finding is broadly consistent with a previous study of healthy term-born neonates in which day 1 blood BDNF levels were similar to cord blood levels but had increased by day 4.[79] Different immune cells synthesize, store, and release BDNF, and increased plasma levels of BDNF are associated with a variety of immune responses, as alluded to earlier. Hence, Malamitsi-Puchner and colleagues[107] suggested that the day 1 spike in blood BDNF in term and preterm infants may reflect an immune response to antigenic stimuli, induced by the sudden transition from the intrauterine to the extrauterine environment. However, these investigators point out that although this possibly protective response is maintained in the term neonates, it is largely lost in the preterm infants by day 4 and may contribute to their neurodevelopmental vulnerability.

More recently, Rao and colleagues[108] measured serial changes in blood BDNF from birth (ie, cord blood) to 60 days in slightly more premature infants born at 27.4 $\pm$ 2.1 weeks' GA. Cord blood BDNF was comparable with that in the preterm infants in the study by Malamitsi-Puchner and colleagues.[107] By day 6, blood BDNF had returned to cord blood levels and continued to increase progressively until day 60, although it changed little between days 30 and 60. However, mean blood BDNF in these preterm infants at day 60[108] was only around 65% of the levels recorded in term-born infants at days 1 and 4.[107] Furthermore, blood BDNF at day 60 was low in those infants who went on to develop retinopathy of prematurity (ROP), and lower still in those infants requiring surgery for stage 3 or higher ROP than those who did not. This finding suggests a close relationship between cortical BDNF levels and the experience-dependent development of visual function. However, we are not aware of any studies examining cord blood and postnatal circulating BDNF levels with motor outcomes in either preterm or term-born infants. Overall, these findings suggest prematurity is associated with reduced BDNF abundance and associated with certain adverse neurologic outcomes in the preterm infant.

If an important factor determining the likelihood of a good neuromotor outcome in preterm infants is whether or not they have abnormally low BDNF production and abundance, the question then is "Can we increase BDNF abundance in the preterm infant therapeutically?" One approach is the administration of exogenous BDNF and the other is to use strategies that increase endogenous levels of BDNF. We have briefly mentioned animal-based research showing the beneficial effects of exogenous administration of BDNF on neurologic outcomes in neonatal rats after hypoxic-ischemic insult. We are not aware of any similar research in human neonates, although there is considerable interest in the use of BDNF in treatment of neuropathologic conditions in the adult, such as Parkinson disease, stroke, and spinal cord injury, and in neuropsychiatric disorders such as depression (reviewed in Ref.[104]). The main challenge to using exogenous BDNF as a treatment is finding a method of delivery that overcomes the blood-brain barrier, penetrates to the deeper brain layers instead of only superficially, concomitantly limits the effect area to avoid possible adverse effects, and one that can be used chronically.[104] Therefore, the most feasible option is to increase endogenous BDNF levels; there is increasing evidence that this strategy might be possible through enriched environments, including regular physical exercise.

Enriched Environments

There is a wealth of data from animal studies showing that enriched environments are associated with morphologic changes in the brain, including increases in dendritic spine density, neuronal numbers, and neuroplastic capacity[109–111] (reviewed in Ref.[112]). In animal studies, environmental enrichment usually refers to adding features to home cages (toys, exploratory tunnels, social and family groups) to stimulate and facilitate sensory, cognitive, and motor functioning in addition to that offered by standard housing. Although environmental enrichment seems to have positive effects on neurologic functioning at all ages, the animal studies imply that if individuals are exposed to an environmental enrichment before adulthood there may be additional positive effects on the developing brain.[113] Similarly, we recently reported that in term-born but low birthweight adult humans, experiencing an early postnatal environment with less socioeconomic disadvantage and having an educated mother partly ameliorates the reduced motor cortex excitability and lower educational achievement associated with poor fetal growth.[49] It is not yet clear which elements of an enriched environment underlie the changes in neuroplasticity, but a critical component in all models seems to be physical activity.

Rodents with access to a running wheel for voluntary exercise develop higher BDNF levels in certain parts of the brain, including the hippocampus.[100,114] In humans, increased motor activity increases brain BDNF levels,[115,116] and individuals who undergo regular physical exercise have a greater capacity for experimental motor neuroplasticity induction than their age-matched sedentary peers.[117] Low BDNF levels in old age are associated with increased frailty,[118] but a physical therapy intervention consisting of a 10-week progressive dynamic resistance-training program of 60 minutes' duration performed 3 times a week resulted in significantly increased circulating BDNF that correlated with functional improvement, irrespective of the level of the participant's frailty before the program.[118] Rodent studies show that increased motor activity has positive effects on neurologic outcomes other than alterations in BDNF, including increasing angiogenesis and microglia number in rat cortex, and increasing neuronal proliferation and survival in the hippocampus (reviewed in Ref.[113]).

Increased motor activity alone may be beneficial in improving some brain morphology and neuroplasticity, but the animal studies show that it does not account for all of the behavioral, cognitive, and cellular change associated with an enriched environment.[113] However, there is increasing evidence to suggest that regular physical activity may be a more important component in improving the preterm child's overall neurodevelopmental outcome than previously believed. Considerable future research is required to determine what the components that constitute an enriched environment for the preterm child are.

DEVELOPMENTAL CARE APPROACHES AND MOTOR OUTCOMES

In terms of the influence of developmental care interventions on motor development, the most recent Cochrane review[119] reported "very limited evidence of a long-term positive effect" of NIDCAP on motor outcomes at 5 years corrected age. However, analysis of the effectiveness of developmental care interventions is hampered by several study design issues. Of the 36 studies in Symington and Pinelli's systematic review,[119] none met all of the methodological quality criteria. In particular, allocation concealment was absent or inadequate in 26 of the 36 studies. The key role of allocation concealment in randomized controlled trials (RCTs) is to blind those responsible for allocating participants to treatment or control groups from rerouting participants with a better prognosis to the treatment group and those with a worse prognosis to the control group, thereby biasing the outcome in favor of the treatment.[120] Unlike other RCTs using drugs versus placebo, or similar, it is impossible to blind the care providers during developmental care RCTs. This situation should not preclude blinding of those assessing the neurodevelopmental outcomes in the infants. However, only half of the 36 studies included had clear blinding of the outcomes assessors, and only 17 showed clear evidence of complete follow-up.[119]

Blauw-Hospers and Hadders-Algra[121] recently suggested that part of the problem in assessing the efficacy of early interventions such as NIDCAP may be that the outcome measures used (predominantly Bayley Scales of Infant Development and Griffiths Developmental Scales) lack the sensitivity to detect small improvements in motor development that nonetheless have a significant effect on the infant's future motor function. Based on their systematic analysis Blauw-Hospers and Hadders-Algra[121] also suggested that the type of intervention of benefit to preterm neonates differs from the type of intervention most beneficial for infants at term age or older, so the infant age at which the effectiveness of an intervention is assessed is also likely to be critical. Interventions that mimic the intrauterine environment and minimize stress seem best for preterm infants, whereas after term-equivalent age, specific motor training and activities that stimulate a child's engagement in a range of active motor behaviors is most effective.[121]

We currently lack a good body of methodologically sound RCTs on the various preterm developmental care interventions, and have too few data on postterm motor development programs for sound critical analysis. In addition, perhaps we should also reconsider how we care for late preterm infants, both in terms of identifying those most at risk of a suboptimal neurodevelopmental outcome and in providing evidence-based proactive interventions in infancy. The current approach is generally relatively ad hoc and reactive, often occurring later in childhood once a child's developmental dysfunction has become obvious.

SUMMARY

Damage to the developing motor system is still the most common injury seen in preterm infants. Despite advances in knowledge and technology, we are still unable to accurately predict the likely neuromotor outcome for most preterm infants.

Although a general rule of thumb might be that children with no perinatal history of brain lesions are likely to have the best outcome, this first presupposes that the infant has undergone some form of imaging to enable diagnosis, and that the imaging techniques used were able to detect any existing injury. Emerging evidence suggests that there are a significant number of preterm children with more subtle neurophysiologic abnormalities that are not detected in the neonatal period, and that a significant proportion of these children are late preterm. The main reasons for this are likely to be twofold. First, we are just beginning to have the techniques at our disposal either to identify microstructural abnormalities or to assess the developing neurophysiology painlessly or adequately. Second, until recently the prevailing view was that late preterm infants are by and large neurologically normal or within normal limits, but although the late preterm tend not to require NICU or special care, they are nonetheless are at greater risk of a poorer neuromotor and cognitive outcome than their term-born peers.

Preterm birth alters brain growth trajectories during a time of rapid growth and this perturbed growth results in aberrant connectivity between brain regions. Data from TMS studies suggest that this aberrant connectivity is still evident in early adolescence. Minimizing stress in the preterm infant may have multiple neurologic effects including not adding to aberrant connectivity and reducing the likelihood of programming abnormal stress responsiveness. This situation in turn may help preserve existing neuroplastic capacity. This finding not only has implications for NICU care of high-risk infants but also for educating parents of late preterm infants who are discharged soon after birth. However, well-designed, well-powered RCTs of the short-term and long-term efficacy of early intervention strategies on preterm infants at all ages are required.

The motor areas of the human brain seem to contribute to some higher cognitive functions, and strategies designed to optimize neuromotor development and neuroplastic capacity in children born preterm are likely to be important in optimizing their cognitive development. The motor areas are still highly plastic in early adolescence, suggesting the window of opportunity is wider than previously believed, although the evidence regarding educational, behavioral, and social difficulties in school-age children strongly suggests that intervention must start early in childhood.

REFERENCES

1. Hack M, Fanaroff AA. Outcomes of children of extremely low birthweight and gestational age in the 1990s. Semin Neonatol 2000;5(2):89–106.
2. Bracewell M, Marlow N. Patterns of motor disability in very preterm children. Ment Retard Dev Disabil Res Rev 2002;8(4):241–8.
3. Davis NM, Ford GW, Anderson PJ, et al. Developmental coordination disorder at 8 years of age in a regional cohort of extremely-low-birthweight or very preterm infants. Dev Med Child Neurol 2007;49(5):325–30.
4. Holsti L, Grunau RV, Whitfield MF. Developmental coordination disorder in extremely low birth weight children at nine years. J Dev Behav Pediatr 2002; 23(1):9–15.
5. Jongmans M, Mercuri E, de Vries L, et al. Minor neurological signs and perceptual-motor difficulties in prematurely born children. Arch Dis Child Fetal Neonatal Ed 1997;76(1):F9–14.
6. Powls A, Botting N, Cooke RWI, et al. Motor impairment in children 12 to 13 years old with a birthweight of less than 1250 g. Arch Dis Child Fetal Neonatal Ed 1995;73(2):F62–6.

7. Sullivan MC, McGrath MM. Perinatal morbidity, mild motor delay, and later school outcomes. Dev Med Child Neurol 2003;45(2):104–12.
8. Jain L. School outcome in late preterm infants: a cause for concern. J Pediatr 2008;153(1):5–6.
9. Jobe AH. A new disease–the late preterm infant. J Pediatr 2008;153(1):A1.
10. Kramer MS. Late preterm birth: appreciable risks, rising incidence. J Pediatr 2009;154(2):159–60.
11. Hanakawa T. Rostral premotor cortex as a gateway between motor and cognitive networks. Neurosci Res 2011;70(2):144–54.
12. Cisek P, Kalaska JF. Neural correlates of mental rehearsal in dorsal premotor cortex. Nature 2004;431(7011):993–6.
13. Abe M, Hanakawa T. Functional coupling underlying motor and cognitive functions of the dorsal premotor cortex. Behav Brain Res 2009;198(1):13–23.
14. Billiards SS, Pierson CR, Haynes RL, et al. Is the late preterm infant more vulnerable to gray matter injury than the term infant? Clin Perinatol 2006;33(4):915–33.
15. Volpe JJ. Brain injury in premature infants: a complex amalgam of destructive and developmental disturbances. Lancet Neurol 2009;8(1):110–24.
16. Johnston MV, Fatemi A, Wilson MA, et al. Treatment advances in neonatal neuroprotection and neurointensive care. Lancet Neurol 2011;10(4):372–82.
17. Kapellou O, Counsell SJ, Kennea N, et al. Abnormal cortical development after premature birth shown by altered allometric scaling of brain growth. PLoS Med 2006;3(8):e265.
18. Peterson BS. Brain imaging studies of the anatomical and functional consequences of preterm birth for human brain development. Ann N Y Acad Sci 2003;1008:219–37.
19. Peterson BS, Anderson AW, Ehrenkranz R, et al. Regional brain volumes and their later neurodevelopmental correlates in term and preterm infants. Pediatrics 2003;111(5):939–48.
20. Peterson BS, Vohr B, Staib LH, et al. Regional brain volume abnormalities and long-term cognitive outcome in preterm infants. JAMA 2000;284(15):1939–47.
21. van Soelen ILC, Brouwer RM, Peper JS, et al. Effects of gestational age and birth weight on brain volumes in healthy 9 year-old children. J Pediatr 2010;156(6):896–901.
22. Kesler SR, Ment LR, Vohr B, et al. Volumetric analysis of regional cerebral development in preterm children. Pediatr Neurol 2004;31(5):318–25.
23. Ajayi-Obe M, Saeed N, Cowan FM, et al. Reduced development of cerebral cortex in extremely preterm infants. Lancet 2000;356(9236):1162–3.
24. Counsell SJ, Edwards AD, Chew AT, et al. Specific relations between neurodevelopmental abilities and white matter microstructure in children born preterm. Brain 2008;131(12):3201–8.
25. Myers EH, Hampson M, Vohr B, et al. Functional connectivity to a right hemisphere language center in prematurely born adolescents. Neuroimage 2010;51(4):1445–52.
26. Smyser CD, Inder TE, Shimony JS, et al. Longitudinal analysis of neural network development in preterm infants. Cereb Cortex 2010;20(12):2852–62.
27. Smyser CD, Snyder AZ, Neil JJ. Functional connectivity MRI in infants: exploration of the functional organization of the developing brain. Neuroimage 2011;56(3):1437–52.
28. Schafer RJ, Lacadie C, Vohr B, et al. Alterations in functional connectivity for language in prematurely born adolescents. Brain 2009;132(3):661–70.

29. Eyre JA, Miller S, Clowry GJ, et al. Functional corticospinal projections are established prenatally in the human foetus permitting involvement in the development of spinal motor centres. Brain 2000;123(Pt 1):51–64.

30. Eyre J, Miller S, Clowry GJ. The development of the corticospinal tract in humans. In: Pascual Leone D, Davey G, Wasserman EM, et al, editors. Handbook of transcranial magnetic stimulation. London: Arnold; 2002. p. 235–50.

31. Lemon RN. Descending pathways in motor control. Annu Rev Neurosci 2008; 31(1):195–218.

32. Eyre JA. Developmental plasticity of the corticospinal system. In: Boniface S, Ziemann U, editors. Plasticity in the human brain: investigations with transcranial magnetic brain stimulation. Cambridge (United Kingdom): Cambridge University Press; 2003. p. 62–89.

33. O'Sullivan MC, Miller S, Ramesh V, et al. Abnormal development of biceps brachii phasic stretch reflex and persistence of short latency heteronymous reflexes from biceps to triceps brachii in spastic cerebral palsy. Brain 1998;121(12):2381–95.

34. Skranes J, Vangberg TR, Kulseng S, et al. Clinical findings and white matter abnormalities seen on diffusion tensor imaging in adolescents with very low birth weight. Brain 2007;130(3):654–66.

35. Kinney HC. The near-term (late preterm) human brain and risk for periventricular leukomalacia: a review. Optimizing Care and Outcomes for Late Preterm (Near-Term) Infants Part 2. Semin Perinatol 2006;30(2):81–8.

36. Petersen NC, Butler JE, Taylor JL, et al. Probing the corticospinal link between the motor cortex and motoneurones: some neglected aspects of human motor cortical function. Acta Physiol 2010;198(4):403–16.

37. Kumar A, Juhasz C, Asano E, et al. Diffusion tensor imaging study of the cortical origin and course of the corticospinal tract in healthy children. AJNR Am J Neuroradiol 2009;30(10):1963–70.

38. Kloppel S, Baumer T, Kroeger J, et al. The cortical motor threshold reflects microstructural properties of cerebral white matter. Neuroimage 2008;40(4): 1782–91.

39. Bengtsson SL, Nagy Z, Skare S, et al. Extensive piano practicing has regionally specific effects on white matter development. Nat Neurosci 2005;8(9):1148–50.

40. Koh TH, Eyre JA. Maturation of corticospinal tracts assessed by electromagnetic stimulation of the motor cortex. Arch Dis Child 1988;63(11):1347–52.

41. Thomas JE, Lambert EH. Ulnar nerve conduction velocity and H-reflex in infants and children. J Appl Physiol 1960;15(1):1–9.

42. Desmedt JE, Brunko E, Debecker J. Maturation of the somatosensory evoked potentials in normal infants and children, with special reference to the early N1 component. Electroencephalogr Clin Neurophysiol 1976;40(1):43–58.

43. Fallang B, Oien I, Hellem E, et al. Quality of reaching and postural control in young preterm infants is related to neuromotor outcome at 6 years. Pediatr Res 2005;58(2):347–53.

44. Gardosi J, Figueras F, Clausson B, et al. The customised growth potential: an international research tool to study the epidemiology of fetal growth. Paediatr Perinat Epidemiol 2011;25(1):2–10.

45. Customised centile calculator–grow-centile [computer program]. Version 5.1: gestation network. 2006. Available at: http://www.gestation.net/. Accessed May 17, 2011.

46. Pitcher JB, Higgins RD, Burns NR, et al. Gestation length and fetal growth have independent effects on corticospinal development in children: the PREMOCODE study. Clin Neurophysiol 2010;121(Suppl 1):S169.

47. Henderson SE, Sugden DA, Barnett AL. Movement assessment battery for children–examiners manual. 2nd edition. London: Pearson Assessment; 2007.

48. Nagy Z, Westerburg H, Skare S, et al. Preterm children have disturbances of white matter at 11 years of age as shown by diffusion tensor imaging. Pediatr Res 2003;54(5):672–9.

49. Pitcher JB, Robertson AL, Cockington RA, et al. Prenatal growth and early postnatal influences on adult motor cortical excitability. Pediatrics 2009;124(1):e128–36.

50. Pitcher JB, Schneider LA, Drysdale JL, et al. Gestation length and fetal growth have different effects on corticospinal excitability and motor skill development in children. J Dev Orig Health Dis 2011;2(1):S10.

51. Marlow N, Roberts BL, Cooke RW. Motor skills in extremely low birthweight children at the age of 6 years. Arch Dis Child 1989;64(6):839–47.

52. Marlow N, Roberts L, Cooke R. Outcome at 8 years for children with birth weights of 1250 g or less. Arch Dis Child 1993;68(3 Spec No):286–90.

53. Chyi LJ, Lee HC, Hintz SR, et al. School outcomes of late preterm infants: special needs and challenges for infants born at 32 to 36 weeks gestation. J Pediatr 2008;153(1):25–31.

54. Huddy CLJ, Johnson A, Hope PL. Educational and behavioural problems in babies of 32-35 weeks gestation. Arch Dis Child Fetal Neonatal Ed 2001; 85(1):F23–8.

55. Kirkegaard I, Obel C, Hedegaard M, et al. Gestational age and birth weight in relation to school performance of 10-year-old children: a follow-up study of children born after 32 completed weeks. Pediatrics 2006;118(4):1600–6.

56. Meister IG, Weier K, Staedtgen M, et al. Covert word reading induces a late response in the hand motor system of the language dominant hemisphere. Neuroscience 2009;161(1):67–72.

57. Meister IG, Wilson SM, Deblieck C, et al. The essential role of premotor cortex in speech perception. Curr Biol 2007;17(19):1692–6.

58. Raposo A, Moss HE, Stamatakis EA, et al. Modulation of motor and premotor cortices by actions, action words and action sentences. Neuropsychologia 2009;47(2):388–96.

59. Roy A, Craighero L, Fabbri Destro M, et al. Phonological and lexical motor facilitation during speech listening: a transcranial magnetic stimulation study. J Physiol Paris 2008;102(1–3):101–5.

60. Fadiga L, Craighero L, Buccino G, et al. Speech listening specifically modulates the excitability of tongue muscles: a TMS study. Eur J Neurosci 2002;15(2): 399–402.

61. Flöel A, Ellger T, Breitenstein C, et al. Language perception activates the hand motor cortex: implications for motor theories of speech perception. Eur J Neurosci 2003;18(3):704–8.

62. Fazio P, Cantagallo A, Craighero L, et al. Encoding of human action in Broca's area. Brain 2009;132(7):1980–8.

63. Knecht S, Drager B, Deppe M, et al. Handedness and hemispheric language dominance in healthy humans. Brain 2000;123(12):2512–8.

64. Pitcher JB, Henderson-Smart DJ, Robinson JS. Prenatal programming of human motor function. Adv Exp Med Biol 2006;573:41–57.

65. Tolsa CB, Zimine S, Warfield SK, et al. Early alteration of structural and functional brain development in premature infants born with intrauterine growth restriction. Pediatr Res 2004;56(1):132–8.

66. Lodygensky GA, Seghier ML, Warfield SK, et al. Intrauterine growth restriction affects the preterm infant's hippocampus. Pediatr Res 2008;3(4):438–43.

67. Martinussen M, Fischl B, Larsson HB, et al. Cerebral cortex thickness in 15-year-old adolescents with low birth weight measured by an automated MRI-based method. Brain 2005;128(11):2588–96.
68. Martinussen M, Flanders DW, Fischl B, et al. Segmental brain volumes and cognitive and perceptual correlates in 15-year-old adolescents with low birth weight. J Pediatr 2009;155(6):848–53.e841.
69. Harding JE, McCowan LM. Perinatal predictors of growth patterns to 18 months in children born small for gestational age. Early Hum Dev 2003;74(1):13–26.
70. Casey PH, Whiteside-Mansell L, Barrett K, et al. Impact of prenatal and/or post-natal growth problems in low birth weight preterm infants on school-age outcomes: an 8-year longitudinal evaluation. Pediatrics 2006;118(3):1078–86.
71. Leitner Y, Fattal-Valevski A, Geva R, et al. Neurodevelopmental outcome of children with intrauterine growth retardation: a longitudinal, 10-year prospective study. J Child Neurol 2007;22(5):580–7.
72. Yeung MY. Postnatal growth, neurodevelopment and altered adiposity after preterm birth–from a clinical nutrition perspective. Acta Paediatr 2006;95(8):909–17.
73. Latal-Hajnal B, von Siebenthal K, Kovari H, et al. Postnatal growth in VLBW infants: significant association with neurodevelopmental outcome. J Pediatr 2003;143(2):163–70.
74. Dabydeen L, Thomas JE, Aston TJ, et al. High-energy and -protein diet increases brain and corticospinal tract growth in term and preterm infants after perinatal brain injury. Pediatrics 2008;121(1):148–56.
75. Lumbers ER, Yu ZY, Gibson KJ. The selfish brain and the barker hypothesis. Clin Exp Pharmacol Physiol 2001;28(11):942–7.
76. Baschat AA, Hecher K. Fetal growth restriction due to placental disease. Semin Perinatol 2004;28(1):67–80.
77. Pitcher JB, Riley AM, Ridding MC. Children born preterm have reduced long term depression (LTD)-like neuroplasticity. J Dev Orig Health Dis 2011;2(1):S145.
78. Ridding MC, Rothwell JC. Is there a future for therapeutic use of transcranial magnetic stimulation? Nat Rev Neurosci 2007;8(7):559–67.
79. Nikolaou KE, Malamitsi-Puchner A, Boutsikou T, et al. The varying patterns of neurotrophin changes in the perinatal period. Ann N Y Acad Sci 2006;1092(1):426–33.
80. Davis EP, Waffarn F, Sandman CA. Prenatal treatment with glucocorticoids sensitizes the hpa axis response to stress among full-term infants. Dev Psychobiol 2011;53(2):175–83.
81. Phillips DI. Programming of the stress response: a fundamental mechanism underlying the long-term effects of the fetal environment? J Intern Med 2007;261(5):453–60.
82. Sullivan MC, Hawes K, Winchester SB, et al. Developmental origins theory from prematurity to adult disease. J Obstet Gynecol Neonatal Nurs 2008;37(2):158–64.
83. Kajantie E, Feldt K, Raikkonen K, et al. Body size at birth predicts hypothalamic-pituitary-adrenal axis response to psychosocial stress at age 60 to 70 years. J Clin Endocrinol Metab 2007;92(11):4094–100.
84. Bettendorf M, Albers N, Bauer J, et al. Longitudinal evaluation of salivary cortisol levels in full-term and preterm neonates. Horm Res 1998;50(6):303–8.
85. Nykanen P, Raivio T, Heinonen K, et al. Circulating glucocorticoid bioactivity and serum cortisol concentrations in premature infants: the influence of exogenous glucocorticoids and clinical factors. Eur J Endocrinol 2007;156(5):577–83.

86. Buyukkayhan D, Ozturk MA, Kurtoglu S, et al. Effect of antenatal betamethasone use on adrenal gland size and endogenous cortisol and 17-hydroxyprogesterone in preterm neonates. J Pediatr Endocrinol Metab 2009;22(11):1027–31.

87. Fernandez EF, Montman R, Watterberg KL. ACTH and cortisol response to critical illness in term and late preterm newborns. J Perinatol 2008;28(12):797–802.

88. Grunau RE, Haley DW, Whitfield MF, et al. Altered basal cortisol levels at 3, 6, 8 and 18 months in infants born at extremely low gestational age. J Pediatr 2007; 150(2):151–6.

89. Anand KJ. Pain, plasticity, and premature birth: a prescription for permanent suffering? Nat Med 2000;6:971–3.

90. Grunau RE, Holsti L, Haley DW, et al. Neonatal procedural pain exposure predicts lower cortisol and behavioral reactivity in preterm infants in the NICU. Pain 2005;113(3):293–300.

91. Grunau RE, Weinberg J, Whitfield MF. Neonatal procedural pain and preterm infant cortisol response to novelty at 8 months. Pediatrics 2004;114(1):e77–84.

92. Als H, Lawhon G, Duffy FH, et al. Individualized developmental care for the very low-birth-weight preterm infant. JAMA 1994;272(11):853–8.

93. Nyqvist KH, Anderson GC, Bergman N, et al. Towards universal Kangaroo Mother Care: recommendations and report from the First European conference and Seventh International Workshop on Kangaroo Mother Care. Acta Paediatr 2010;99(6):820–6.

94. Sale MV, Ridding MC, Nordstrom MA. Cortisol inhibits neuroplasticity induction in human motor cortex. J Neurosci 2008;28(33):8285–93.

95. Haley DW, Grunau RE, Weinberg J, et al. Physiological correlates of memory recall in infancy: vagal tone, cortisol, and imitation in preterm and full-term infants at 6 months. Infant Behav Dev 2010;33(2):219–34.

96. Harris A, Seckl J. Glucocorticoids, prenatal stress and the programming of disease. Horm Behav 2011;59(3):279–89.

97. Thomason ME, Yoo DJ, Glover GH, et al. BDNF genotype modulates resting functional connectivity in children. Front Hum Neurosci 2009;3:55.

98. Chan JR, Cosgaya JM, Wu YJ, et al. Inaugural article: neurotrophins are key mediators of the myelination program in the peripheral nervous system. Proc Natl Acad Sci U S A 2001;98(25):14661–8.

99. Lu B, Gottschalk W. Modulation of hippocampal synaptic transmission and plasticity by neurotrophins. In: Seil FJ, editor, Progress in brain research, vol. 128. Elsevier; 2000. p. 231–41.

100. Mattson MP, Maudsley S, Martin B. BDNF and 5-HT: a dynamic duo in age-related neuronal plasticity and neurodegenerative disorders. Trends Neurosci 2004;27(10):589–94.

101. Almli CR, Levy TJ, Han BH, et al. BDNF protects against spatial memory deficits following neonatal hypoxia-ischemia. Exp Neurol 2000;166(1):99–114.

102. Han BH, Holtzman DM. BDNF protects the neonatal brain from hypoxic-ischemic injury in vivo via the ERK pathway. J Neurosci 2000;20(15):5775–81.

103. Cheng Y, Gidday JM, Yan Q, et al. Marked age-dependent neuroprotection by brain-derived neurotrophic factor against neonatal hypoxic–ischemic brain injury. Ann Neurol 1997;41(4):521–9.

104. Nagahara AH, Tuszynski MH. Potential therapeutic uses of BDNF in neurological and psychiatric disorders. Nat Rev Drug Discov 2011;10(3):209–19.

105. Chouthai NS, Sampers J, Desai N, et al. Changes in neurotrophin levels in umbilical cord blood from infants with different gestational ages and clinical conditions. Pediatr Res 2003;53(6):965–9.

106. Ringstedt T, Linnarsson S, Wagner J, et al. BDNF regulates reelin expression and Cajal-Retzius cell development in the cerebral cortex. Neuron 1998;21(2): 305–15.

107. Malamitsi-Puchner A, Economou E, Rigopoulou O, et al. Perinatal changes of brain-derived neurotrophic factor in pre- and fullterm neonates. Early Hum Dev 2004;76(1):17–22.

108. Rao R, Mashburn CB, Mao J, et al. Brain-derived neurotrophic factor in infants <32 weeks gestational age: correlation with antenatal factors and postnatal outcomes. Pediatr Res 2009;65(5):548–52.

109. Leggio MG, Mandolesi L, Federico F, et al. Environmental enrichment promotes improved spatial abilities and enhanced dendritic growth in the rat. Behav Brain Res 2005;163(1):78–90.

110. Gelfo F, De Bartolo P, Giovine A, et al. Layer and regional effects of environmental enrichment on the pyramidal neuron morphology of the rat. Neurobiol Learn Mem 2009;91(4):353–65.

111. Goshen I, Avital A, Kreisel T, et al. Environmental enrichment restores memory functioning in mice with impaired IL-1 signaling via reinstatement of long-term potentiation and spine size enlargement. J Neurosci 2009; 29(11):3395–403.

112. Petrosini L, De Bartolo P, Foti F, et al. On whether the environmental enrichment may provide cognitive and brain reserves. Brain Res Rev 2009;61(2):221–39.

113. Nithianantharajah J, Hannan AJ. Enriched environments, experience-dependent plasticity and disorders of the nervous system. Nat Rev Neurosci 2006;7(9): 697–709.

114. Tong L, Shen H, Perreau VM, et al. Effects of exercise on gene-expression profile in the rat hippocampus. Neurobiol Dis 2001;8(6):1046–56.

115. Neeper SA, Gómez-Pinilla F, Choi J, et al. Physical activity increases mRNA for brain-derived neurotrophic factor and nerve growth factor in rat brain. Brain Res 1996;726(1–2):49–56.

116. Gustafsson G, Lira CM, Johansson J, et al. The acute response of plasma brain-derived neurotrophic factor as a result of exercise in major depressive disorder. Psychiatry Res 2009;169(3):244–8.

117. Cirillo J, Lavender AP, Ridding MC, et al. Motor cortex plasticity induced by paired associative stimulation is enhanced in physically active individuals. J Physiol 2009;587(24):5831–42.

118. Coelho FM, Pereira DS, Lustosa LP, et al. Physical therapy intervention (PTI) increases plasma brain-derived neurotrophic factor (BDNF) levels in non-frail and pre-frail elderly women. Arch Gerontol Geriatr 2011, 10.1016/j.archger. 2011.05.014.

119. Symington AJ, Pinelli J. Developmental care for promoting development and preventing morbidity in preterm infants. Cochrane Database Syst Rev 2006; 19(2).

120. Schulz KF. Assessing allocation concealment and blinding in randomised controlled trials: why bother? Evid Based Med 2000;5(2):36–8.

121. Blauw-Hospers CH, Hadders-Algra M. A systematic review of the effects of early intervention on motor development. Dev Med Child Neurol 2005;47(6):421–32.

The Gustatory and Olfactory Systems During Infancy: Implications for Development of Feeding Behaviors in the High-Risk Neonate

Sarah V. Lipchock, PhD, Danielle R. Reed, PhD,
Julie A. Mennella, PhD*

KEYWORDS

- High-risk neonate • Gustatory system development
- Olfactory system development • Infant feeding behaviors
- Flavor learning

Our senses of taste and smell are intimately connected to nutrition and allow us to reject those foods that are harmful and to seek out those that are beneficial and pleasurable.[1] During the past several decades, researchers have begun to unravel some of the mysteries underlying the ontogeny of the function of these senses as well as the roles they play in food choice, health, and social interactions.

Building on the scientific definition of flavor and the basic biology of taste and smell, we summarize insights gleaned from basic scientific research in the chemical senses, with a focus on the sensory capabilities of the human infant and the inherent contributions of genetic differences in taste perception and the plasticity of the chemical senses in the development of flavor and food preferences. We highlight differences between normal and high-risk neonates with regard to early sensory experiences and their potential impact on learning and later feeding.

Preparation of this manuscript was supported in part by grant DC011287 and training grant T32-DC00014-32 from the National Institute of Deafness and Other Communication Disorders and by grant HD37119 from the Eunice Kennedy Shriver National Institute of Child Health and Human Development. The content is solely the responsibility of the authors and does not necessarily represent the official views of the National Institutes of Health.
Monell Chemical Senses Center, 3500 Market Street, Philadelphia, PA 19104-3308, USA
* Corresponding author.
E-mail address: mennella@monell.org

Clin Perinatol 38 (2011) 627–641
doi:10.1016/j.clp.2011.08.008
0095-5108/11/$ – see front matter

DEFINITION OF FLAVOR

Flavor, a powerful determinant of human ingestion throughout the life span, is a product of several sensory systems, most notably those of the chemical senses, taste and smell. The perceptions arising from these 2 senses are often confused and misappropriated.[2] Sensations such as garlic, chocolate, anise, and lemon are erroneously attributed to the taste system per se, when only a few primary taste qualities can be perceived by the tongue: sweet, salty, bitter, sour, and savory. On the other hand, smell sensations encompass thousands of diverse qualities, including the flavors noted earlier. As illustrated in **Fig. 1**, the receptors for the olfactory system, located high in the nasal chambers, are stimulated not only during inhalation (orthonasal route) but also when infants suck and when children and adults swallow, as chemical constituents in foods and beverages reach the nasal receptors by passing from the oral cavity through the nasal pharynx (retronasal route). It is this retronasal stimulation arising from the molecules of foodstuffs that leads to the predominant flavor sensations.

BASIC FLAVOR BIOLOGY

Taste occurs when chemicals come into contact with taste receptors on the tongue, palate, throat, epiglottis, or esophagus that then send signals to the brain. Taste receptor cells are the interface between the oral environment and the nervous system (reviewed in Ref.[3]). These cells, arranged in groups of 50 to 100 to form taste buds, contain the proteins necessary to recognize each of the 5 types of taste: sweet, salty, sour, bitter, and savory. Salty and sour foods are recognized by ion channels.[4] Salty taste is most commonly imparted by sodium ions in sodium chloride, but other sodium and nonsodium salts also convey a salty characteristic. Sour taste is generated by protons in acids. Sweet, bitter, and savory tastes are translated to the brain via G-protein-coupled receptors (GPCRs): type I GPCRs (T1R1, T1R2, and T1R3) are stimulated by sweet (T1R2 + T1R3) and savory (T1R1 + T1R3) compounds,[5,6] whereas bitter compounds are recognized by type II GPCRs (T2Rs).[7,8] T2Rs recognize a variety of unpleasant-tasting compounds and may have evolved as a warning to avoid toxins.[9,10]

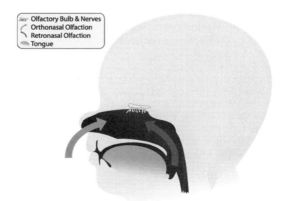

Fig. 1. Orthonasal (*green arrow*) and retronasal (*purple arrow*) routes of olfaction.

Odors are recognized by olfactory receptors, which are located on a small patch of tissue in the nasal cavity. Olfactory receptors are GPCRs that are generated by the largest mammalian gene superfamily, with more than 400 functional genes.[11,12] The olfactory system becomes tuned to respond to stimuli in different ways based on the experience of the individual and the context in which odors are experienced.[13,14] Olfactory signals combine with taste signals to communicate flavor to the brain.[15,16]

GENETICS OF FLAVOR

Polymorphisms in the genes that encode taste and odorant receptors result in differential sensory patterns in humans, by altering amino acid sequences of receptors, which alters their function, or by altering gene expression.[17–28] Although these mutations are found in a variety of receptor genes, few examples have been well characterized in the literature.

Polymorphisms in the bitter taste receptor gene *TAS2R38* are the most studied of all taste receptor variants. Genetic variation in this receptor translates into individual differences in taste sensitivity for the synthetic compounds phenylthiocarbamide and propylthiouracil (PROP), as well as bitter-tasting compounds commonly found in cruciferous vegetables.[29] The polymorphisms result in changes to the amino acid sequence of the receptor from alanine-valine-isoleucine (AVI) in nontasters to proline-alanine-valine (PAV) in tasters.[17,30,31] These polymorphisms allow homozygous AVI people to enjoy broccoli or turnips without perceiving the bitterness that heterozygous AVI/PAV and especially homozygous PAV people taste.[32] Studies in children and their mothers indicate that the phenotype-genotype relationship for PROP sensitivity varies with age, such that AVI/PAV heterozygous children are more sensitive to PROP than are heterozygous adults, with adolescents being intermediate.[25,33] These results imply that within the same genotype, taste sensitivity can change over the life span (from more to less bitter sensitivity).

A commonly cited example of individual variation in human olfaction is the perception of androstenone, a volatile steroid found in human perspiration, boar saliva, some pork products, truffles, and celery.[34] Whereas some individuals describe this volatile as "sweaty and urinous," others perceive it as smelling "sweet and floral," or odorless.[35–37] The odorant receptor *OR7D4* is activated by androstenone, and recently 2 polymorphisms were identified within the gene that change the amino acid sequence and impair the function of the receptor.[21] Individuals with the arginine-threonine variant smell androstenone, and those with the tryptophan-methionine variant find it to be odorless. Similar to bitterness sensitivity, the ability to detect androstenone seems to change with age.[38–40]

EXTRAORAL TASTE AND NUTRIENT SENSING

Although not much is known about their function, taste receptors have been found in many extraoral tissues, including the lungs, brain, gut, and reproductive system.[41–44] Sweet and bitter receptors are both found in the gut but have different functions. Sweet receptors regulate local glucose transporters to enhance glucose uptake,[45] whereas 1 function of the bitter taste receptors is to regulate the absorption of toxic secondary plant compounds or other poisons.[46] Bitter receptors are also found in the upper and lower airways in mammals,[47–50] and they are probably also present in humans. Their function in the airway is not known, but 1 possibility is that they bitter molecules secreted by bacteria and may evoke immune or other responses to clear the airway of pathogens.[51] The developmental trajectory of extraoral bitter and sweet receptors in gut, airway, and other tissues is not known, either in humans or in other species.

PRENATAL AND POSTNATAL DEVELOPMENT OF FLAVOR

Both olfactory and taste receptors must be functional in order for a human fetus or infant to sense flavor. The primary olfactory receptors are formed by the eighth week of gestation (see Ref.[52] for a review) and are functional as early as the 24th week.[53,54] Taste cells also begin to form at 7 to 8 weeks of gestation[55,56]; by 13 to 15 weeks they look like mature receptor cells, and by around 17 weeks they are considered functionally mature. Fetal swallowing begins at approximately 12 weeks of gestation.[57,58] Around 18 weeks, gestational nonnutritive suckling begins, and the sucking and swallowing actions are coordinated by 35 to 40 weeks of gestation. Near the end of gestation the fetus swallows significant amounts of amniotic fluid. After 6 months of gestation, when the epithelial plugs no longer obstruct the air passages, amniotic fluid is also inhaled. The inhalation and swallowing of amniotic fluid are the first chemosensory experiences of the fetus and mark the beginning of flavor learning.

Amniotic fluid, the first food of infants, contains a wide range of nutrients that have particular tastes, such as glucose, fructose, lactic acid, fatty acids, and amino acids,[59] as well as the flavors (for which the odors are perceived retronasally) of the foods consumed by the mother.[60,61] The fetus can detect these tastes and flavors: fetal swallowing frequency increases in response to the introduction of sweet solutions into the amniotic fluid and decreases in response to the introduction of bitter solutions[59,62]; this observation may be one of the first indications that our basic biology favors consumption of sweet tastes and avoidance of bitter tastes.

A similar response pattern is seen shortly after birth: within hours and days of being born, young infants react as would be expected to pleasurable and aversive taste stimuli[63–72]; provision of sweet or savory solutions to neonates elicits rhythmical tongue protrusions, lip smacks, lip and finger sucking, and elevation of the corners of the mouth, all of which have been interpreted as a positive or hedonic response.[71,72] In contrast, neonates gape, wrinkle their noses, shake their heads, flail their arms, and frown in response to a bitter solution.[63,72] Concentrated sour solutions elicit lip pursing and, to a certain extent, gaping, nose wrinkling, and arm flailing, as well as tongue protrusions and lip smacking.[63,72,73] Unlike the other basic tastes, salt taste receives a neutral reaction from neonates; the taste for salt does not emerge until later in infancy and then remains throughout childhood and adolescence.[74]

These specific affective reactions to differing taste stimuli are strikingly similar across cultures[68,73,75] and species,[72,76–79] suggesting a basic biologic underpinning for the flavors and foods youngsters prefer and avoid. The convergence of research findings supports the conclusion that the innate preference for sweets and rejection of bitter tastes in humans are consequences of selection, favoring consumption of high-energy, vitamin-rich fruit and vegetable diets and avoidance of bitter, poisonous fruits and plants. Thus, when we examine children's dietary patterns from the perspective of the development of taste, the foods children naturally prefer (eg, sweet snacks) and those they dislike (eg, bitter-tasting green vegetables) are not surprising and reflect their basic biology.

In addition to containing chemicals with distinct taste properties, amniotic fluid contains volatile chemicals (flavors) transmitted from the maternal diet,[60,61,80] which, by at least the second trimester, seem to be detected by the fetus. Shortly after birth, infants respond differently to flavors experienced in amniotic fluid, indicating that memories are formed from these early sensory experiences. For example, neonates whose mothers consumed an anise-flavored beverage or ate garlic-containing foods throughout pregnancy were more accepting of and interested in (as measured by mouthing and orienting) anise and garlic odors.[80,81] Similar findings were observed with alcohol odors.[82]

Learning about the dietary choices of the mother continues when infants experience the flavors of the mother's diet transmitted in breast milk. Young mammals first learn about the dietary choices of their mothers through transmitted flavor cues, a type of learning documented in a wide variety of species (see Ref.[83] for review). Following from this finding, researchers determined that many flavors (eg, anise, garlic, ethanol, carrot, mint, vanilla, blue cheese) pass from mother to offspring through breast milk.[60,61,83–86] Human infants detect the flavors in mother's milk, as evidenced by changes in their suckling rate, patterning and duration of feeding and intake,[60,85,86] and differential acceptance of similarly flavored foods at weaning and beyond.[60,87–89] Similarly, breastfed infants were more accepting of fruits and vegetables than were formula-fed infants, but only if their mothers regularly ate these foods themselves.[87]

That these early flavor experiences can influence the acceptance of foods was first shown in a randomized, controlled study of mothers who consumed carrot juice for several days each week during the last trimester of pregnancy or for a similar period during the first 3 months of lactation.[88] The control group drank water and avoided carrots and carrot juice during both pregnancy and lactation. When mothers weaned their infants around 6 months of age, the children were tested for acceptance of plain cereal on 1 day and carrot-flavored cereal on another. Infants who experienced the flavor of carrots in either amniotic fluid or mother's milk responded more favorably (eg, ate more, made fewer faces of distaste) to carrot-flavored cereal than did nonexposed control infants. Thus, as with many other mammals, human infants' prenatal and postnatal experiences with food flavors transmitted from the mother's diet lead to greater acceptance and enjoyment of these foods during weaning.

SENSITIVE PERIOD FOR FLAVOR LEARNING

Although the types of flavors that breastfed infants experience before their first taste of solid foods reflect the culinary practices of their mothers, which varies from infant to infant,[60,87] formula-fed infants are usually exposed to constant flavors after birth and before weaning, because most formula-fed infants experience a single type of formula.[90] The absence of a robust experimental paradigm, like that used for other sensory systems (eg, vision, audition/language) and in other animals, has inhibited progress in understanding whether human flavor programming shows age-related changes in functional plasticity, commonly referred to as sensitive periods. To address this gap, a model system was used that exploits the naturally occurring flavor variation in infant formulas.[91,92]

In the United States, formulas are available for healthy term infants and for special medical purposes (such as preterm infants or infants with inborn errors of metabolism). Among the formulas for healthy term infants, one of the main distinctions is their protein source or degree of protein hydrolysis. Cow milk formula (CMF) is the most common formula consumed by infants, accounting for 76% of all US infant formula sales in 2000.[93] Its protein usually includes combinations of intact casein and whey proteins.[94,95] Extensive protein hydrolysate formula (ePHF), a type of formula typically fed to infants who have cow milk protein allergy or intolerance to intact protein, is less prevalent in use than is CMF.[93] The milk proteins (ie, whey, casein) in ePHF are treated with enzymes to break down the protein structure to reduce allergenicity; these formulas contain low-molecular-weight peptides and free amino acids. Partial protein hydrolysate formulas (pPHF) contain whey or casein milk proteins that are enzymatically treated but to a lesser extent than for ePHF. The varying composition and degree of hydrolysis among hydrolysate formulas affect formula flavor profiles.[96] To adults who were not fed ePHF during infancy, it is extremely unpalatable compared with CMF because of the distinctive, unpleasant flavors of PHF, including both volatile (odors) and nonvolatile (eg, bitter and sour tastes) components.

Using the flavor differences between CMF and ePHF as a model system, a window of acceptance was identified during which young infants readily accept ePHF. Beginning around 4 months of age and continuing through adulthood, its flavor is rejected unless the individual was exposed to ePHF earlier in life (consistent with anecdotal pediatrician reports that it is difficult to begin feeding ePHF to infants aged 4 or more months). Thus, depending on an individual's exposure to its flavor during the first few months of life, ePHF acquires a different hedonic tone, or perceived pleasantness.[91]

A randomized trial was conducted to begin to characterize the effects of the timing and duration of early-life exposure when hedonic responses to PHF flavors are established. Infants were randomized to be fed ePHF for 1 month beginning at 1.5 months, 2.5 months, or 3.5 months, or for 3 months beginning at 1.5 months.[92] All groups were then compared with control groups that had either no ePHF exposure or 7 months of ePHF exposure. At 7.5 months, infant acceptance of ePHF was tested with complete meals of both formulas. Among infants who began feeding ePHF at 1.5 months, those fed for 1 month were as accepting of ePHF as those fed for 3 months. That is, flavor experience of a brief occurrence (1 month) before the baby is 3.5 months of age is sufficient to maintain acceptance. However, infants fed ePHF for 1 month were less accepting than infants exposed to ePHF for the entire 7 months. Early exposure is also important: infants exposed to ePHF for 1 month starting at 3.5 months were less accepting of ePHF at 7.5 months of age than were infants exposed at an earlier age. Maternal perceptions of infants' enjoyment of the formulas and the frequency of facial expressions of distaste were consistent with both the exposure-related and timing-related differences in intake. Early exposure eliminated the age-related rejection seen in unexposed infants and resulted in a complete shift in hedonic tone.[92]

The effects of early exposure to ePHF are persistent, leading to heightened preferences for the taste and aroma of ePHF and foods containing similar volatiles or tastes (eg, bitter, sour, and savory) at weaning and several years after children's last exposure to the formula. Children fed ePHF had an increased preference for sour-flavored apple juice[75,97] and savory-tasting, bitter-tasting, sour-tasting and plain cereals compared with other children.[98] The mothers of these children were also more likely to list broccoli as one of their child's preferred vegetables than were mothers of infants fed CMF.[97]

Why should there be a sensitive period in the early acceptance of the flavor of ePHF? First, presuming there is an adaptive reason, it clearly has nothing directly to do with hydrolyzed protein formulas, which were introduced only a half-century ago. These observations with formulas may conveniently expose a more fundamental aspect of early mammalian flavor learning. We hypothesize that it is important for the human infant to accept and be particularly (but not exclusively) attracted to the flavors that are consumed by the culture and, more specifically, by the mother. All else being equal, these are the flavors that are associated with nutritious foods or, at least, foods the mother has access to, and the foods and flavors that the infant will experience at weaning and probably thereafter. Under this hypothesis, much of the normal exposure would occur in utero and during breastfeeding, because flavors mothers consume are transferred to these chemosensory environments. Additional research is needed to determine the extent to which early exposure (and the lack of early exposure) to these flavors, perhaps during sensitive periods of development, helps establish enduring preferences for foods and flavors.

CHALLENGES FOR THE HIGH-RISK NEONATE

The first few months of life are an essential part of the flavor learning process for humans, and during this period the sensory experiences of the high-risk neonate are drastically different from those of a typical infant, lacking continuity with prenatal sensory experiences. Preterm infants are often unable to coordinate sucking, swallowing, and breathing, so nasogastric or orogastric tube feeding is used to provide adequate nutrition.[99] When fed by a tube, infants likely have a relatively constrained olfactory and flavor experience in the context of feeding because their nutrition bypasses the oral and nasal cavities. Even those who are tube fed human milk may not have the opportunity to experience retronasally the flavors present in milk. Furthermore, it is unknown how the body responds when nutrients are sensed in the gut but have not been sensed in the oral cavity.

Tube-fed infants increase nonnutritive sucking when exposed to the smell of mother's milk through an infant olfactometer, suggesting that exposure to maternal nutrient odor may assist in transition to oral feeding.[100] However, in the neonatal intensive care unit and normal infant wards in hospitals, infants are also exposed to (and learn about) unpleasant or noxious odors, including disinfectants, antibacterial compounds, and cleaning solutions.[101] The long-term consequences of this altered sensory environment remain unknown.

Tube feeding is generally performed using either preterm formula or fortified human milk.[102–104] Greater efforts are being made to increase the amount of human milk given to preterm infants because human milk provides many benefits such as improved immune status and increased cognitive development, whereas successful expression of breast milk allows for more maternal involvement in feeding and increases maternal confidence.[105–119] We hypothesize that, given the presence of functional taste receptors in both the oral cavity and the gut,[45] increasing intake of human milk is beneficial for future feeding behavior because the extraoral stimulation of milk on gut taste receptors may aid in the transition from tube feeding to breastfeeding. Encouraging the mother to pump breast milk also increases the likelihood that the child will eventually be able to transition to the breast and experience the flavors in mother's milk within the sensitive window for flavor learning.[106]

In addition to altered oral sensory exposure, infants who are tube fed do not have early experience with traditional feeding behaviors (sucking, swallowing, and chewing). However, there has been a paucity of experimental research in this area on how such altered sensory experiences affect later behaviors associated with feeding. Several case studies from the 1960s revealed that if children were not introduced to solid foods at the time when they are first able to chew, acceptance of these foods became difficult.[120] In 3 of the cases, the children had esophageal atresia and were tube fed beginning days after birth. Repair of the esophagus did not happen until 16 to 22 months later, at which point 2 of the 3 patients readily accepted fluids, but all 3 had significant difficulty transitioning to solid food. Long-term tube feeding may affect the physical development of feeding behaviors, with consequences lasting into childhood.

When tube feeding occurs for a short period (15–20 days), in combination with nonnutritive sucking, infants generally transition well to oral feeding.[121–124] However, if the tube feeding lasts for a longer period (>45 days), it becomes more difficult for the child to make the transition. In a study of 9 infants who were tube fed for at least 2 months starting from birth, the infants refused all attempts at oral feeding and reacted with agitation, arching, tongue thrusting, gagging, and vomiting.[124] The infants also had an absent or deficient sucking reflex and a gag reflex that was triggered by any foreign object. To help wean the children, during tube feedings at regular intervals the infants were provided with stimulation to reproduce normal feeding as closely as possible. They were cradled in their mother's arms, the gums and palate were massaged, and the tongue was stimulated with breast milk from the mother's finger to stimulate the sucking reflex. Eight of the children eventually weaned from tube to oral feeding, with those who were tube fed the longest requiring the most time to establish normal eating behavior. The investigators of the study hypothesize that stimulation during tube feeding helps inhibit the gag reflex, creates an association among tactile, olfactory, and taste sensations and the mechanical replenishing of the stomach, and establishes normal circadian rhythms.[124]

High-risk infants are also faced with a wide array of medical conditions that contribute to temporary or permanent alteration of taste and smell as adults. Many medications, including antibiotics and antiinflammatory agents, have been shown to alter taste and smell, and these are commonly given to high-risk neonates.[125–127] Feeding problems can lead to vitamin deficiencies, which have also been linked to altered taste and smell.[128] Gastroesophageal reflux disease is another common problem in preterm infants and results in a sour or bitter taste in the mouth from reflux of stomach acid up the esophagus and into the throat.[129] The long-term effects of these alterations on the development of flavor preferences in the child are not known.

CONCLUDING REMARKS

Every culture differs in the flavor principles that characterize its cuisine and the types of foods preferred by the families who identify with its traditions. Thus, cultural traditions guide the types of food individuals eat on a daily basis. Although many would argue that learning about these flavor principles, food preferences, and cultural traditions begins when parents serve their children cultural meals during family dinners, research shows that this learning begins long before a child ever consumes solid food. Flavors of the mother's diet are transmitted to the offspring through the amniotic fluid and breast milk, and infants more readily accept flavors that they have already experienced through these 2 media when fed as solid foods at weaning. The recent discoveries of taste receptors in tissues outside the oral cavity add to the complexity of this system. Infants may also be sensing bitter stimuli in the airways or sweet stimuli in the gut, and the development of these sensory systems is not yet understood.

Because the senses of taste and smell are the major determinants of whether young children accept a food (eg, they eat only what they like), these senses take on greater significance in understanding the biologic basis for children's food choices. Not being exposed to the flavors of healthy foods early in life can have detrimental consequences. Although there are innate responses to the basic tastes, and some individuals may be more sensitive to some tastes because of genotype, the development of these chemical senses has inherent plasticity that interacts with early-life experiences to shape and modify flavor and food preferences. Such functional plasticity, one of the main characteristics of the brain, highlights the ability to change behavior based on experience. Our biology is not necessarily our destiny.

Although we are beginning to learn how the chemical senses develop during infancy and their impact on food choices and other behaviors, there are many gaps in our knowledge. In particular, we know little about the contingencies for early learning and how the absence of early postnatal chemosensory experience (eg, absence of breast-feeding), disruptions in mother-infant attachment (eg, tube feeding of high-risk infants), or negative associations with early feeding (eg, chemical smells in hospital settings) interfere with the acquisition of feeding skills. The increasing awareness of the importance of infant feeding behavior makes it imperative to determine the extent to which restoration of normal oral motor and sensory experiences affect feeding behavior and nutrition.

More research is needed to develop evidence-based practices aimed at infant feeding difficulties, which constitute a medically and economically important complication for some neonatal diseases. Applying the knowledge gleaned from such research and clinical practice, which takes into account the developing sensory world of the child, could have long-term consequences in preventing eating disorders in early infancy. Moreover, understanding the development and functioning of these senses may assist in the development of evidence-based strategies to improve children's diets, because many of the illnesses that plague modern society (eg, obesity, diabetes, and hypertension) are often the consequence of poor food choices that start in childhood.

REFERENCES

1. Reed DR, Knaapila A. Genetics of taste and smell: poisons and pleasures. Prog Mol Biol Transl Sci 2010;94:213–40.
2. Rozin P. "Taste-smell confusions" and the duality of the olfactory sense. Percept Psychophys 1982;31(4):397–401.
3. Breslin PA, Spector AC. Mammalian taste perception. Curr Biol 2008;18(4): R148–55.
4. Medler K, Kinnamon S. Transduction mechanisms in taste cells. In: Frings S, Bradley J, editors. Transduction channels in sensory cells. Weinheim (Germany): Wiley-VCH; 2004. p. 153–74.
5. Zhao GQ, Zhang Y, Hoon MA, et al. The receptors for mammalian sweet and umami taste. Cell 2003;115(3):255–66.
6. Li X, Staszewski L, Xu H, et al. Human receptors for sweet and umami taste. Proc Natl Acad Sci U S A 2002;99(7):4692–6.
7. Chandrashekar J, Mueller KL, Hoon MA, et al. T2Rs function as bitter taste receptors. Cell 2000;100(6):703–11.
8. Adler E, Hoon MA, Mueller KL, et al. A novel family of mammalian taste receptors. Cell 2000;100(6):693–702.
9. Peyrot des Gachons C, Beauchamp GK, Stern RM, et al. Bitter taste induces nausea. Curr Biol 2011;21(7):R247–8.
10. Fox AL. The relationship between chemical constitution and taste. Proc Natl Acad Sci U S A 1932;18(1):115–20.
11. Buck L, Axel R. A novel multigene family may encode odorant receptors: a molecular basis for odor recognition. Cell 1991;65(1):175–87.
12. Hasin-Brumshtein Y, Lancet D, Olender T. Human olfaction: from genomic variation to phenotypic diversity. Trends Genet 2009;25(4):178–84.
13. Epple G, Herz RS. Ambient odors associated to failure influence cognitive performance in children. Dev Psychobiol 1999;35(2):103–7.
14. Forestell CA, Mennella JA. Children's hedonic judgments of cigarette smoke odor: effects of parental smoking and maternal mood. Psychol Addict Behav 2005;19(4):423–32.

15. Small DM, Gerber JC, Mak YE, et al. Differential neural responses evoked by orthonasal versus retronasal odorant perception in humans. Neuron 2005;47(4): 593–605.

16. Bender G, Hummel T, Negoias S, et al. Separate signals for orthonasal vs. retronasal perception of food but not nonfood odors. Behav Neurosci 2009;123(3): 481–9.

17. Bufe B, Breslin PA, Kuhn C, et al. The molecular basis of individual differences in phenylthiocarbamide and propylthiouracil bitterness perception. Curr Biol 2005; 15(4):322–7.

18. Chen QY, Alarcon S, Tharp A, et al. Perceptual variation in umami taste and polymorphisms in TAS1R taste receptor genes. Am J Clin Nutr 2009;90(3): 770S–9S.

19. Eriksson N, Macpherson JM, Tung J, et al. Web-based, participant-driven studies yield novel genetic associations for common traits. PLoS Genet 2010; 6(6):e1000993.

20. Fushan AA, Simons CT, Slack JP, et al. Allelic polymorphism within the TAS1R3 promoter is associated with human taste sensitivity to sucrose. Curr Biol 2009; 19(15):1288–93.

21. Keller A, Zhuang H, Chi Q, et al. Genetic variation in a human odorant receptor alters odour perception. Nature 2007;449(7161):468–72.

22. Kim UK, Breslin PA, Reed D, et al. Genetics of human taste perception. J Dent Res 2004;83(6):448–53.

23. Kim UK, Wooding S, Riaz N, et al. Variation in the human TAS1R taste receptor genes. Chem Senses 2006;31(7):599–611.

24. Menashe I, Abaffy T, Hasin Y, et al. Genetic elucidation of human hyperosmia to isovaleric acid. PLoS Biol 2007;5(11):e284.

25. Mennella JA, Pepino MY, Reed DR. Genetic and environmental determinants of bitter perception and sweet preferences. Pediatrics 2005;115(2): e216–22.

26. Pelchat ML, Bykowski C, Duke FF, et al. Excretion and perception of a characteristic odor in urine after asparagus ingestion: a psychophysical and genetic study. Chem Senses 2011;36(1):9–17.

27. Reed DR, Zhu G, Breslin PA, et al. The perception of quinine taste intensity is associated with common genetic variants in a bitter receptor cluster on chromosome 12. Hum Mol Genet 2010;19(21):4278–85.

28. Shigemura N, Shirosaki S, Ohkuri T, et al. Variation in umami perception and in candidate genes for the umami receptor in mice and humans. Am J Clin Nutr 2009;90(3):764S–9S.

29. Wooding S, Gunn H, Ramos P, et al. Genetics and bitter taste responses to goitrin, a plant toxin found in vegetables. Chem Senses 2010;35(8): 685–92.

30. Kim UK, Jorgenson E, Coon H, et al. Positional cloning of the human quantitative trait locus underlying taste sensitivity to phenylthiocarbamide. Science 2003; 299(5610):1221–5.

31. Timpson NJ, Heron J, Day IN, et al. Refining associations between TAS2R38 diplotypes and the 6-n-propylthiouracil (PROP) taste test: findings from the Avon Longitudinal Study of Parents and Children. BMC Genet 2007;8:51.

32. Sandell MA, Breslin PA. Variability in a taste-receptor gene determines whether we taste toxins in food. Curr Biol 2006;16(18):R792–4.

33. Mennella JA, Pepino MY, Duke FF, et al. Age modifies the genotype-phenotype relationship for the bitter receptor TAS2R38. BMC Genet 2010;11:60.

34. Wysocki CJ, Dorries KM, Beauchamp GK. Ability to perceive androstenone can be acquired by ostensibly anosmic people. Proc Natl Acad Sci U S A 1989; 86(20):7976–8.

35. Pollack MS, Wysocki CJ, Beauchamp GK, et al. Absence of HLA association or linkage for variations in sensitivity to the odor of androstenone. Immunogenetics 1982;15(6):579–89.

36. Theimer ET, Yoshida T, Klaiber EM. Olfaction and molecular shape. Chirality as a requisite for odor. J Agric Food Chem 1977;25(5):1168–77.

37. Wysocki CJ, Beauchamp GK. Ability to smell androstenone is genetically determined. Proc Natl Acad Sci U S A 1984;81(15):4899–902.

38. Bekaert KM, Tuyttens FA, Duchateau L, et al. The sensitivity of Flemish citizens to androstenone: influence of gender, age, location and smoking habits. Meat Sci 2011;88(3):548–52.

39. Dorries KM, Schmidt HJ, Beauchamp GK, et al. Changes in sensitivity to the odor of androstenone during adolescence. Dev Psychobiol 1989;22(5):423–35.

40. Wysocki CJ, Gilbert AN. National Geographic Smell Survey. Effects of age are heterogenous. Ann N Y Acad Sci 1989;561:12–28.

41. Ren X, Zhou L, Terwilliger R, et al. Sweet taste signaling functions as a hypothalamic glucose sensor. Front Integr Neurosci 2009;3:12.

42. Behrens M, Meyerhof W. Oral and extraoral bitter taste receptors. Results Probl Cell Differ 2010;52:87–99.

43. Iwatsuki K, Nomura M, Shibata A, et al. Generation and characterization of T1R2-LacZ knock-in mouse. Biochem Biophys Res Commun 2010;402(3): 495–9.

44. Kokrashvili Z, Mosinger B, Margolskee RF. T1r3 and alpha-gustducin in gut regulate secretion of glucagon-like peptide-1. Ann N Y Acad Sci 2009;1170: 91–4.

45. Margolskee RF, Dyer J, Kokrashvili Z, et al. T1R3 and gustducin in gut sense sugars to regulate expression of Na+-glucose cotransporter 1. Proc Natl Acad Sci U S A 2007;104(38):15075–80.

46. Jeon TI, Seo YK, Osborne TF. Gut bitter taste receptor signaling induces ABCB1 through a mechanism involving CCK. Biochem J 2011;438(1):33–7.

47. Finger TE, Bottger B, Hansen A, et al. Solitary chemoreceptor cells in the nasal cavity serve as sentinels of respiration. Proc Natl Acad Sci U S A 2003;100(15): 8981–6.

48. Gulbransen BD, Clapp TR, Finger TE, et al. Nasal solitary chemoreceptor cell responses to bitter and trigeminal stimulants in vitro. J Neurophysiol 2008; 99(6):2929–37.

49. Deshpande DA, Wang WC, McIlmoyle EL, et al. Bitter taste receptors on airway smooth muscle bronchodilate by localized calcium signaling and reverse obstruction. Nat Med 2010;16(11):1299–304.

50. Tizzano M, Cristofoletti M, Sbarbati A, et al. Expression of taste receptors in solitary chemosensory cells of rodent airways. BMC Pulm Med 2011;11:3.

51. Tizzano M, Gulbransen BD, Vandenbeuch A, et al. Nasal chemosensory cells use bitter taste signaling to detect irritants and bacterial signals. Proc Natl Acad Sci U S A 2010;107:3210–5.

52. Ganchrow JR, Mennella JA. The ontogeny of human flavor perception. In: Doty RL, editor. Handbook of olfaction and gustation, 2nd edition. 2nd edition. New York: Marcel Dekker; 2003. p. 823–946.

53. Chuah MI, Zheng DR. Olfactory marker protein is present in olfactory receptor cells of human fetuses. Neuroscience 1987;23(1):363–70.

54. Johnson EW, Eller PM, Jafek BW. Distribution of OMP-, PGP 9.5- and CaBP-like immunoreactive chemoreceptor neurons in the developing human olfactory epithelium. Anat Embryol (Berl) 1995;191(4):311–7.

55. Bradley RM, Stern IB. The development of the human taste bud during the foetal period. J Anat 1967;101(Pt 4):743–52.

56. Witt M, Reutter K. Scanning electron microscopical studies of developing gustatory papillae in humans. Chem Senses 1997;22(6):601–12.

57. Pritchard JA. Deglutition by normal and anencephalic fetuses. Obstet Gynecol 1965;25:289–97.

58. Schaffer JP. The lateral wall of the cayum nasi in man with special reference to the various developmental stages. J Morphol 1910;21:613–7.

59. Liley AW. Disorders of amniotic fluid. In: Assali NS, editor. Pathophysiology of gestation. Fetal placental disorders. New York: Academic Press; 1972. p. 157–206.

60. Mennella JA, Jagnow CP, Beauchamp GK. Prenatal and postnatal flavor learning by human infants. Pediatrics 2001;107(6):E88.

61. Mennella JA, Johnson A, Beauchamp GK. Garlic ingestion by pregnant women alters the odor of amniotic fluid. Chem Senses 1995;20(2):207–9.

62. DeSnoo K. Das trinkende Kind im Uterus. Monoats Geburtsh Gynaekol 1937; 105:88–97 [in German].

63. Desor JA, Maller O, Andrews K. Ingestive responses of human newborns to salty, sour, and bitter stimuli. J Comp Physiol Psychol 1975;89(8):966–70.

64. Beauchamp GK, Pearson P. Human development and umami taste. Physiol Behav 1991;49(5):1009–12.

65. Desor JA, Maller O, Greene LS. Preference for sweet in humans: infants, children and adults. In: Weiffenbach JM, editor. Taste and development: the genesis of sweet preference. Washington, DC: Government Printing Office; 1977. p. 161–73.

66. Fox NA, Davidson RJ. Taste-elicited changes in facial signs of emotion and the asymmetry of brain electrical activity in human newborns. Neuropsychologia 1986;24(3):417–22.

67. Maller O, Desor JA. Effect of taste on ingestion by human newborns. Symp Oral Sens Percept 1973;(4):279–91.

68. Rosenstein D, Oster H. Differential facial responses to four basic tastes in newborns. Child Dev 1988;59(6):1555–68.

69. Steiner JE. The gustofacial response: observation on normal and anencephalic newborn infants. Symp Oral Sens Percept 1973;(4):254–78.

70. Steiner JE. The human gustofacial response. In: Bosma JF, editor. Fourth symposium of oral sensation and perception: development in the fetus and infant. Bethesda (MD): Department of Health, Education and Welfare; 1973. p. 254–78.

71. Steiner JE. What the human neonate can tell us about umami. In: Kawamura Y, Kare MR, editors. Umami: a basic taste. New York: Marcel Dekker; 1987. p. 97–123.

72. Steiner JE, Glaser D, Hawilo ME, et al. Comparative expression of hedonic impact: affective reactions to taste by human infants and other primates. Neurosci Biobehav Rev 2001;25(1):53–74.

73. Steiner JE. Facial expressions of the neonate infant indicating the hedonics of food related chemical stimuli. In: Weiffenbach JM, editor. Taste and development: the genesis of sweet preference. Washington, DC: Government Printing Office; 1977. p. 173–89.

74. Beauchamp GK, Cowart BJ, Moran M. Developmental changes in salt acceptability in human infants. Dev Psychobiol 1986;19(1):17–25.
75. Liem DG, Mennella JA. Sweet and sour preferences during childhood: role of early experiences. Dev Psychobiol 2002;41(4):388–95.
76. Brining SK, Belecky TL, Smith DV. Taste reactivity in the hamster. Physiol Behav 1991;49(6):1265–72.
77. Ganchrow JR, Steiner JE, Bartana A. Behavioral reactions to gustatory stimuli in young chicks (*Gallus gallus domesticus*). Dev Psychobiol 1990;23(2):103–17.
78. Grill HJ, Roitman MF, Kaplan JM. A new taste reactivity analysis of the integration of taste and physiological state information. Am J Physiol 1996;271(3 Pt 2):R677–87.
79. Beauchamp GK, Mason JR. Comparative hedonics of taste. In: Bolles RC, editor. The hedonics of taste. Hillsdale (NJ): Lawrence Erlbaum Associates; 1991. p. 159–83.
80. Schaal B, Marlier L, Soussignan R. Human foetuses learn odours from their pregnant mother's diet. Chem Senses 2000;25(6):729–37.
81. Hepper PG. Adaptive fetal learning: prenatal exposure to garlic affects personal preferences. Anim Behav 1988;36:935–6.
82. Faas AE, Sponton ED, Moya PR, et al. Differential responsiveness to alcohol odor in human neonates: effects of maternal consumption during gestation. Alcohol 2000;22(1):7–17.
83. Mennella JA. The chemical senses and the development of flavor preferences in humans. In: Hale TW, Hartmann PE, editors. Textbook on human lactation. Amarillo (TX): Hale Publishing; 2007. p. 403–14.
84. Mennella JA, Beauchamp GK. Maternal diet alters the sensory qualities of human milk and the nursling's behavior. Pediatrics 1991;88(4):737–44.
85. Mennella JA, Beauchamp GK. The transfer of alcohol to human milk. Effects on flavor and the infant's behavior. N Engl J Med 1991;325(14):981–5.
86. Mennella JA, Beauchamp GK. The effects of repeated exposure to garlic-flavored milk on the nursling's behavior. Pediatr Res 1993;34(6):805–8.
87. Forestell CA, Mennella JA. Early determinants of fruit and vegetable acceptance. Pediatrics 2007;120(6):1247–54.
88. Mennella JA, Beauchamp GK. Experience with a flavor in mother's milk modifies the infant's acceptance of flavored cereal. Dev Psychobiol 1999;35(3):197–203.
89. Mennella JA, Beauchamp GK. Mothers' milk enhances the acceptance of cereal during weaning. Pediatr Res 1997;41(2):188–92.
90. Nevo N, Rubin L, Tamir A, et al. Infant feeding patterns in the first 6 months: an assessment in full-term infants. J Pediatr Gastroenterol Nutr 2007;45(2):234–9.
91. Mennella JA, Griffin CE, Beauchamp GK. Flavor programming during infancy. Pediatrics 2004;113(4):840–5.
92. Mennella JA, Lukasewycz LD, Castor SM, et al. The timing and duration of a sensitive period in human flavor learning: a randomized trial. Am J Clin Nutr 2011;93(5):1019–24.
93. Oliveira V, Prell M, Smallwood D, et al. Infant Trends in Formula. In: WIC and the retail price of infant formula, FANRR39-1. U.S. Department of Agriculture, Economic Research Service; 2005. p. 26–33.
94. Similac. Abbot Nutrition: Similac Advance EarlyShield product information. Available at:http://abbottnutrition.com/Products/similac-advance-earlyshield. Accessed January 10, 2010.

95. Hennigs JK, Burhenne N, Stahler F, et al. Sweet taste receptor interacting protein CIB1 is a general inhibitor of InsP(3)-dependent Ca(2+)-release in vivo. J Neurochem 2008;106(5):2249–62.

96. Cook DA, Sarett HP. Design of infant formulas for meeting normal and special needs. In: Lifshitz F, editor. Pediatric nutrition: infant feedings, deficiencies, diseases. New York: Marcel Dekker; 1982. p. 71–85.

97. Mennella JA, Beauchamp GK. Flavor experiences during formula feeding are related to preferences during childhood. Early Hum Dev 2002;68(2):71–82.

98. Mennella JA, Forestell CA, Morgan LK, et al. Early milk feeding influences taste acceptance and liking during infancy. Am J Clin Nutr 2009;90(3):780S–8S.

99. Toce SS, Keenan WJ, Homan SM. Enteral feeding in very-low-birth-weight infants. A comparison of two nasogastric methods. Am J Dis Child 1987;141(4):439–44.

100. Bingham PM, Churchill D, Ashikaga T. Breast milk odor via olfactometer for tube-fed, premature infants. Behav Res Methods 2007;39(3):630–4.

101. Laudert S, Liu WF, Blackington S, et al. Implementing potentially better practices to support the neurodevelopment of infants in the NICU. J Perinatol 2007; 27(Suppl 2):S75–93.

102. Heiman H, Schanler RJ. Enteral nutrition for premature infants: the role of human milk. Semin Fetal Neonatal Med 2007;12(1):26–34.

103. Reali A, Greco F, Fanaro S, et al. Fortification of maternal milk for very low birth weight (VLBW) pre-term neonates. Early Hum Dev 2010;86(Suppl 1):33–6.

104. Fanaro S, Ballardini E, Vigi V. Different pre-term formulas for different pre-term infants. Early Hum Dev 2010;86(Suppl 1):27–31.

105. Anderson JW, Johnstone BM, Remley DT. Breast-feeding and cognitive development: a meta-analysis. Am J Clin Nutr 1999;70(4):525–35.

106. Black KA, Hylander MA. Breastfeeding the high risk infant: implications for midwifery management. J Midwifery Womens Health 2000;45(3):238–45.

107. Hylander MA, Strobino DM, Dhanireddy R. Human milk feedings and infection among very low birth weight infants. Pediatrics 1998;102(3):E38.

108. Kavanaugh K, Meier P, Zimmermann B, et al. The rewards outweigh the efforts: breastfeeding outcomes for mothers of preterm infants. J Hum Lact 1997;13(1): 15–21.

109. Lucas A, Cole TJ. Breast milk and neonatal necrotising enterocolitis. Lancet 1990;336(8730):1519–23.

110. Lucas A, Morley R, Cole TJ, et al. Breast milk and subsequent intelligence quotient in children born preterm. Lancet 1992;339(8788):261–4.

111. Meier PP, Brown LP. State of the science. Breastfeeding for mothers and low birth weight infants. Nurs Clin N Am 1996;31(2):351–65.

112. Schanler RJ. Suitability of human milk for the low-birthweight infant. Clin Perinatol 1995;22(1):207–22.

113. Amin SB, Merle KS, Orlando MS, et al. Brainstem maturation in premature infants as a function of enteral feeding type. Pediatrics 2000;106(2 Pt 1):318–22.

114. Bier JA, Oliver T, Ferguson AE, et al. Human milk improves cognitive and motor development of premature infants during infancy. J Hum Lact 2002; 18(4):361–7.

115. Blaymore Bier JA, Oliver T, Ferguson A, et al. Human milk reduces outpatient upper respiratory symptoms in premature infants during their first year of life. J Perinatol 2002;22(5):354–9.

116. Hylander MA, Strobino DM, Pezzullo JC, et al. Association of human milk feedings with a reduction in retinopathy of prematurity among very low birthweight infants. J Perinatol 2001;21(6):356–62.

117. Lucas A, Morley R, Cole TJ. Randomised trial of early diet in preterm babies and later intelligence quotient. BMJ 1998;317(7171):1481–7.
118. Schanler RJ. The use of human milk for premature infants. Pediatr Clin N Am 2001;48(1):207–19.
119. Schanler RJ, Shulman RJ, Lau C. Feeding strategies for premature infants: beneficial outcomes of feeding fortified human milk versus preterm formula. Pediatrics 1999;103(6 Pt 1):1150–7.
120. Illingworth RS, Lister J. The critical or sensitive period, with special reference to certain feeding problems in infants and children. J Pediatr 1964;65:839–48.
121. Bernbaum JC, Pereira GR, Watkins JB, et al. Nonnutritive sucking during gavage feeding enhances growth and maturation in premature infants. Pediatrics 1983;71(1):41–5.
122. Dunbar SB, Jarvis AH, Breyer M. The transition from nonoral to oral feeding in children. Am J Occup Ther 1991;45(5):402–8.
123. Field T, Ignatoff E, Stringer S, et al. Nonnutritive sucking during tube feedings: effects on preterm neonates in an intensive care unit. Pediatrics 1982;70(3): 381–4.
124. Senez C, Guys JM, Mancini J, et al. Weaning children from tube to oral feeding. Childs Nerv Syst 1996;12(10):590–4.
125. Ackerman BH, Kasbekar N. Disturbances of taste and smell induced by drugs. Pharmacotherapy 1997;17(3):482–96.
126. Deems DA, Doty RL, Settle RG, et al. Smell and taste disorders, a study of 750 patients from the University of Pennsylvania Smell and Taste Center. Arch Otolaryngol Head Neck Surg 1991;117(5):519–28.
127. Schiffman SS. Taste and smell losses in normal aging and disease. JAMA 1997; 278(16):1357–62.
128. Goodspeed RB, Gent JF, Catalanotto FA. Chemosensory dysfunction. Clinical evaluation results from a taste and smell clinic. Postgrad Med 1987;81(1): 251–7, 260.
129. Poh CH, Allen L, Malagon I, et al. Riser's reflux–an eye-opening experience. Neurogastroenterol Motil 2010;22(4):387–94.

Infant Bonding and Attachment to the Caregiver: Insights from Basic and Clinical Science

Regina Sullivan, PhD[a],*, Rosemarie Perry, BS[a,b], Aliza Sloan, MA[a], Karine Kleinhaus, MD, MPH[c], Nina Burtchen, MD, MSc[d]

KEYWORDS

• Attachment • Premature infants • Odor • Sensitive period

A common feature of many species is the formation of a mutual attachment between infant and caregiver that ensures that the pair maintains contact. This attachment formation must engage both a maternal behavioral system for provision of care and a behavioral system in the infant that elicits parental care, thus beginning the complex dance of reciprocal attachment. The quality of care received from the mother also programs the infant's emotional and cognitive development by helping to sculpt the developing brain. Because infants must identify their caregivers, a unique pathway for rapid attachment learning seems to support attachment formation, where robust and rapid attachment learning occurs that is akin to the imprinting described for avian species. This occurs in both the mother and the infant, although this review focuses solely on the infant. The characteristics of the infant's attachment to the mother undergo considerable changes as the infant matures into an independent organism.

All authors have no financial disclosures and/or conflicts of interest to disclose.

Funding: NIH MH091451, DC009910, DC003906, and NSF-IOB0850527/0544406 to RMS and NIH MH085807 to KK.

[a] The Emotional Brain Institute, The Nathan S. Kline Institute for Psychiatric Research, Child and Adolescent Psychiatry, New York University School of Medicine, Room 1614, 215 Lexington Avenue, New York, NY 10016, USA

[b] Sackler Graduate Program, Sackler Institute, New York University School of Medicine, 550 First Avenue, New York, NY 10016, USA

[c] Departments of Psychiatry and Environmental Medicine, New York University School of Medicine, 550 First Avenue, New York, NY 10016, USA

[d] Division of Developmental Neuroscience, Department of Psychiatry, Columbia University, 1051 Riverside Drive, New York, NY 10032, USA

* Corresponding author.

E-mail address: regina.sullivan@nyumc.org

Traditionally, the term attachment has been confined to the more complex cognitive, highly specific attachment shown by the time children reach their first birthday.[1,2] This original idea of attachment relates to its theoretical formation and the complex, cognitive representation of the attachment figure seen in older infants and children. However, newborns show specific, highly specialized behavior that can be characterized as attachment or bonding that is influenced by learning and experience. This behavior begins in utero, and adapts to accommodate the changing world as the infant is born and matures. According to this more recent view, high-risk infants, such as premature infants, are vulnerable to forming lower-quality attachments to their caregivers as a result of disrupted critical experience with the mother during prenatal and postnatal development. A better understanding of the complex nature of early-life caregiver-infant relationships may help improve environments and outcomes for at-risk infants.

ATTACHMENT TO THE MOTHER BEGINS IN UTERO

At birth, the full-term infant is attracted to the mother's voice and smell, including the scent of amniotic fluid.[3,4] This attraction to the mother's sensory stimuli is the first sign of the infant's attachment and bonding to the mother. This attachment begins during the last trimester of pregnancy, when auditory and olfactory systems become functional, allowing the fetus to learn about the mother's voice and odors. In the womb the fetus is suspended in amniotic fluid, causing the olfactory mucosa and its receptors to be bathed in waves of this fluid during infant swallowing and thumb sucking. While the uterine acoustic environment is dominated by the rhythmic sound of the mother's blood flow, the mother's voice is carried through her bones and amniotic fluid to the fetal ears.[5] We know that fetal experience with these stimuli is important in shaping the newborn infant's response because experimental manipulation of the amniotic fluid's smell and of sound exposure has profound effects on the newborn's response to these stimuli.[6–8] Based on the animal literature, these stimuli seem to acquire significance through two mechanisms: fetal learning and shaping the development of the fetal brain's sensory systems.[5,9,10]

At birth, these familiar auditory and olfactory stimuli hold particular salience for the infant, as the infant suddenly transitions into a world filled with new sensory experiences, including new sights, sounds, textures, and temperatures. Of course, maternal voice and odors may ease the infant's transition into extrauterine life. A newborn placed on the mother's ventrum will crawl to the mother's breast, as it is not only a potent source of maternal odor but also covered in amniotic fluid and a source of another attractive odor.[11] Even on the first day of life, infants orient to their mother's odor and are soothed, when crying, by their mother's odor.[4,12,13] These behaviors seem to be expressed even in response to the odors of other mothers, but infants show significantly more mouthing to their own mother's odor.[12] In summary, these data suggest that the maternal odor organizes the infant's behavior for nursing.[14] Infants also orient to their mother's voice and will either decrease or increase their sucking rate to hear that voice in an operant conditioning paradigm.[3,15] These infant responses to maternal cues also elicit caregiving from the mother. The mutual infant-caregiver attachment is strengthened during this finely tuned dance of social behaviors as the infant and mother continue to learn about each other.

During the first few days of life, these basic attachment behaviors to the mother change as the infant learns about additional maternal features, such as her face, additional odors, and voice.[3,16–18] The newborn infant prefers the odor of amniotic fluid to breast/maternal odors, although this preference reverses after a week of experience with nursing.[19] Bottle-fed infants show a decreased preference to maternal odors during the first week of life compared with breast-fed infants, perhaps due to their reduced exposure to maternal odors.[7,20] Even bottle-fed infants, however, prefer maternal odors to the odor of formula.[19,21] It should be noted that the caregiver is also learning about the baby. The infant's face, vocalizations, touch, and odor are all rapidly learned by his or her caregiver.[22–26]

Although it is impossible to conclusively determine if infants learn their mother's odors, robust learning has been demonstrated in newborn infants using both sounds[5] and odors.[9] However, this review describes only odor learning. Infants must learn to respond appropriately to their environment by responding to important stimuli while ignoring irrelevant stimuli. Although biological predisposition occurs to some maternal odors because of the odor signature,[27] learning about other aspects of the world and the caregiver is also important.[7,9,28,29] Odor learning and its importance were demonstrated by infant odor preference learning for perfume worn by the mother, which dissipated when the mothers stopped wearing the perfume.[16] This odor learning was also demonstrated in a more controlled classical conditioning experiment.[9] Specifically, infants were presented with a novel odor for 30 seconds with concurrent tactile stimulation similar to a massage or caressing. Standard learning control groups were also included, such as infants who received the odor alone or the odor and massage in a noncontingent manner. One day later the infants, now just 24 to 96 hours old, were given presentations of test odor-only presentations, as a test of learning preference to the odor. Only the infants who had received the odor with concomitant massage showed increased levels of activity and head turns toward the odor, indicating that complex classical conditioning to an odor could occur in newborns. In a more naturalistic experiment, an odor placed in infant bassinets for a day produced a preference for that odor, presumably because of the handling, feeding, and nurturing paired with that odor.[30] Thus, research indicates that infants' exposure to natural or artificial odors can enhance or attenuate their reactive behavior based on postnatal experiences with that odor.

IMPORTANCE OF ATTACHMENT

The critical importance of the mother-infant attachment was noted by Sigmund Freud,[31] who suggested that neuroses in adults were caused by aberrant infant experiences. Our current understanding of the complexity of the infant's first social relationship, however, underwent a paradigm shift in the 1950s. As is documented later, it was the synthesis of research on nonhuman animals and clinical observations of hospitalized and orphaned children who were separated from their mothers that highlighted the critical importance of early-life attachment and its importance for infant mental health.

During the 1950s, clinical observations of orphaned and hospitalized children by Rene Spitz[32] and James Robertson[33] showed detrimental effects of separating the child from the caregiver. Specifically, children expressed extreme emotional distress at separation, which became progressively more depressive-like and subsequently compromised their recovery. This observation of the detrimental effects of caregiver-infant separation initiated a change in hospital visitation policies that enabled parents to visit their children throughout their hospital stay. Within a certain time range and within certain contexts, separating an infant from the mother does not irrevocably damage the infant. As eloquently described in the work of Sir Michael Rutter,[2] maternal deprivation must be viewed not only as a break in a relationship but also as a break in the function of the relationship between the infant and the mother. As noted elsewhere in this review, early life attachment has at least two functions: to keep the baby in the proximity of the mother and to guide brain development. Also, infants frequently have access to other caregivers, such as the father, who can also provide the infant with both the bonding relationship and the sensory stimulation required for normal development.

Concurrent animal work highlighted the role of experience in attachment formation, gradually replacing the notion of attachment as an entirely innate process with a more complex understanding that included a biological predisposition for attachment requiring experience for expression and healthy development. This work showed that the notion of newborns innately knowing their caregiver was too simplistic. Imprinting research in chicks by researchers such as Konrad Lorenz, Niko Tinbergen, and John Hinde first illustrated the importance of experience in attachment formation.[34] At birth, chicks are biologically predetermined to form an attachment, although they have a limited period of time, a critical or sensitive period, in early life when the infant can learn or imprint on their caregiver. The attachment system is straightforward: the chicks attach to the first moving object they see, which under normal circumstances is their mother. The chicks express learned attachment to their caregiver through their following or proximity seeking of the mother. This discovery was an important break-through because it illustrated that there must be a neural circuit for attachment; however, it also indicated that experience plays a critical role in attachment and bonding formation. More recently the neural basis of imprinting, which accounts for both the biological predisposition to attach and the mechanisms underlying the learning aspect of imprinting, has been identified in chicks. These underlying mechanisms involve simplistic brain circuitry, including the dorsocaudal neostriatal complex.[35,36] Although imprinting provides some insight into human attachment, it cannot model all aspects of human attachment and its associated flexibility, resiliency, and children's ability to make bonds with multiple caregivers across longer periods in early childhood.

Additional nonhuman primate research by Harry Harlow and colleagues[37,38] further expanded our understanding of attachment. This work highlighted the organizing function of attachment by showing that disruption of the mother-infant bond disturbs infant emotional and cognitive development. Findings from Harlow's work on infant monkeys appeared to mirror the strong emotional and physical stunting of orphaned and hospitalized infants separated from their mothers. This work emphasized the importance of maternal nurturing of the infant that went beyond food and perfunctory care.

Rodent research in the 1950s also contributed to our understanding of early-life experience and development. Specifically, rodents were provided with different types of sensory stimuli (handling and mild shock), or the infant rodents were separated from their mother. Any of these interventions was capable of dramatically modifying later-life emotionality, such as fear and novelty seeking.[39,40] Stressful stimuli occurring prenatally can also program the earliest maternal behaviors toward the offspring as well as later-life behaviors in the offspring. In one study, when stress hormone was administered to pregnant dams during early gestation the dams displayed altered nursing behaviors, and the newborn pups of treated dams showed decreased juvenile social play and a blunted acoustic startle reflex in adolescence and adulthood, effects that were predicted by frequency of milk ejections in the dams.[41] Together, this research indicates that sensory stimuli and experience alter infant behavior not only directly but also indirectly by altering maternal care.

Thus, findings in various disciplines from humans and other animals began to present a similar story: early-life experience was important for programming emotionality. Through a synthesis of these clinical observations and basic research, a new view of the mother-infant relationship emerged. It was postulated that infants have a biological attachment system that involves learning to identify the caregiver. It also indicated that attachment went beyond the immediate infant-caregiver relationship and highlighted a function of attachment to suggest that the quality of maternal care determines the long-term emotional well-being of the infant. This new view of the mother-infant dyad was facilitated by discussions and meetings of a diverse set of animal researchers and clinicians, and resulted in the paradigm shift, as described earlier, in our understanding of attachment formation.

The psychiatrist John Bowlby[42] had a significant role in integrating this updated view of the mother-infant relationship into our understanding of human attachment, eventually leading to the formulation of his important attachment theory. His interest in human attachment was established as a result of his clinical observations of disturbed children who were deprived of their mothers in childhood. However, his understanding of attachment was also based on the animal models noted earlier and discussions with animal researchers. Specifically, Bowlby's attachment theory suggests that because of the critical importance of attachment for survival, evolution has led children to become biologically preprogrammed to form attachments to their caregiver. Bowlby describes that the attached child exhibits proximity-seeking behavior to the caregiver because the caregiver provides protection and a sense of safety to the child. Once the attachment is formed, the child uses the caregiver as a secure base to explore the world and develop other relationships. Bowlby believed that the child's attachment was built during the first year of life as the child forms a representational mental model of the self and others based on his or her earliest relationship to the mother. Mary Ainsworth,[43] a student and collaborator of John Bowlby, elaborated on his attachment theory and developed the widely used Strange Situation test to characterize attachment quality. This test was developed to define the child's attachment quality. It places the child in a series of 7 increasingly challenging situations (eg, mother ignoring the child, mother leaving the child, and a stranger entering the room), which stressed the child and uncovers disrupted attachment styles uncover possibly disrupted attachment styles. Bowlby's attachment theory and the Strange Situation test greatly increased our understanding of different qualities of attachment and led to a prolific second generation of attachment researchers.

ANIMAL RESEARCH AND EARLY-LIFE EXPERIENCE

Because of ethical concerns the type of research questions one can address in humans is generally limited to correlations while questions of causation can generally be assessed only through the study of disease. Thus, scientists must rely on animal research to access causation and define underlying mechanisms of behaviors, such as attachment, in a more precise and controlled manner. However, the direct translation of animal research to humans requires both caution and an understanding of unique species-specific ecological niches, with a particular awareness of the increasingly complex cognitive processes involved in human attachment relative to other animals.

Nonhuman primates exhibit some aspects of the complex cognitive processes of human attachment and provide an excellent experimental model. Nonhuman primate research by Harlow and Zimmermann[37] and Harlow and Suomi[38] generated clues about the importance of sensory stimulation provided by the mother in producing healthy cognitive and emotional development. For example, a young infant monkey separated from its mother fared better if given access to a tire swing during the separation. However, social interactions with peers, which provide a richer source of sensory stimulation (peer rearing), resulted in even better outcomes, albeit still compromised.[44]

Paradigm-shifting rodent research in the laboratory of Myron Hofer, a psychiatrist interested in a child's bereavement following the death of the caregiver, produced insights into how these sensory stimuli could overcome or repair effects of maternal deprivation.[45] Hofer described the unique role of sensory stimuli from the mother as controlling the behavior, brain, and physiology of rat pups, and suggested that these altered sensory experiences were important for development. The mother was viewed as a hidden regulator of pup behavior and physiology through her sensory stimulation of the pups. By systematically removing and replacing the sensory stimuli normally provided by the mother, he determined that the patterning and intensity of these sensory stimuli were critical for controlling the pup's homeostasis. For example, tactile stimulation from the mother licking or touching the pup increased the excretion of growth hormone, while her warmth increased levels of the neurotransmitter norepinephrine (NE), critical for pups' attachment learning. Other stimuli, such as maternal odor, increased behavioral activity in the pups and indicated that different sensory stimuli singly regulate different behavioral and physiologic systems. Removal of these regulating sensory stimuli, as occurs during separation from the mother, produced dysregulation of the pups' brain functioning and behavior. Hofer further suggested that the short-term effects of maternal separation produce an animal geared to attracting the caregiver, although prolonged separation (ie, long-term removal of the hidden regulators) results in a desynchronization of different physiologic systems depending on the specifics of the separation paradigm (ie, whether other pups are present, whether body temperature is maintained, or whether pups can still smell the maternal odors). Long-term disruptive effects on adult emotionality are the results of physiologic dysregulation, which ultimately produces an animal that does not show adaptive behaviors (ie, inappropriate fear, cognitive impairment, or anxiety). The age and timing of the animal during the experiment produce different long-term outcomes. These effects of maternal behavior on pups include epigenetic changes that are transmitted across generations to continue to control emotionality in the next generation.[46,47]

ANIMAL RESEARCH AND THE NEUROBIOLOGY OF ATTACHMENT

Animal research has facilitated our understanding of human attachment by shedding light on the brain's circuitry used to support attachment. The neural circuit for attachment in children has not been identified and cannot be identified based on the limits of existing technology. Therefore, we must continue to rely on the assumption that a neural circuit in the child's brain supports attachment in the same way as we explore circuitry and neurochemistry in other species. This research has been pivotal in our ability to understand and treat children with attachment disorders and the psychiatric problems that co-occur with these disorders as a result of absent, neglectful, or abusive caregivers. However, much additional animal and human research is still needed.

At present, animal research is helping us characterize infant attachment circuitry in other species, including chicks, rodents, and nonhuman primates. Although it is clear that the circuitry is quite different in avian and mammalian species, a common feature across species is that it is prewired to evoke rapid learning and identification of the caregiver, followed by a unique sequence of infant behaviors designed to elicit caregiving from the mother. In the rodent, the high level of NE in the brain produced during the birth process is physiologically paired with the mother's diet-dependent natural odors to stimulate the learning required for pups to identify and approach their mother and to initiate nursing.[48] This process has been mimicked in the laboratory by substituting maternal odor with artificial odors, such as a peppermint, and injecting the pup with NE to produce an artificial maternal odor that works just as well as natural maternal odor in controlling pups' social interactions with the mother.[49,50] This learned odor has properties powerful enough to produce proximity-seeking behavior in the infant, control pups' social interactions with the mother, and enable nipple attachment for nourishment. The human infant has a surge of NE at birth,[51,52] and it has been speculated that a similar mechanism is used by human infants learning about their mother.[53]

However, as Bowlby observed, children also attach to abusive or neglectful caregivers. The proposed ecological explanation for this seemingly paradoxic attachment is that an infant will attach to his or her caregiver, regardless of the care quality, because the infant's survival depends on that care.[14] The wide phylogenetic representation of attachment to an abusive caregiver includes chicks, rodents, dogs, and nonhuman primates.[54–58]

For example, if an electric shock is administered to a chick during imprinting it still supports learning to follow the surrogate caregiver, although the same stimulus results in avoidance just hours after the critical period for imprinting closes.[55,59] Similarly, administering an electric shock to an infant dog or rat results in a strong attachment to its caregiver.[57,58,60,61] Finally, nonhuman primate and human infants exhibit strong proximity-seeking behavior toward an abusive mother.[62,63]

What, then, is the neurobiological mechanism that allows for aversive or painful stimuli paired with an odor to result in an odor preference? Research on abusive attachment from the authors' laboratory suggests that the lack of plasticity in the infant amygdala may play a leading role,[58] because the amygdala has been shown to be critical for learning fear in adults.[64,65] The amygdala is not activated during attachment learning in the infant rat pup with an abusive caregiver, nor in more controlled classic fear-conditioning experiments where pups learn attachment odors.[57,66,67] This finding suggests that the amygdala is activated neither during social interactions with the mother in infancy nor during encounters with aversive stimuli. These findings have been demonstrated only in infant rats; they are strikingly different from findings in older animals where the amygdala is readily evoked by aversive stimuli as well as during classic fear conditioning.[68–72] This process has been shown in both rodents and humans. In addition, as has been suggested by research in nonhuman primates, the amygdala may not be associated with early-life infant attachment but is involved in social behavior in adulthood.[73,74] Furthermore, work by Tottenham and Sheridan[75] suggests that the child's amygdala is not as readily engaged as the adult amygdala. Together, these data suggest unique attributes of early infancy that support infant attachment: the infant brain is not an immature version of the adult brain but seems to support learning approach responses, while inhibiting learned avoidance responses. This process occurs presumably to ensure that infants approach their caregiver regardless of the quality of care received. However, at least in the rodent, although odor pain conditioning enhances attachment odor in infancy, it is associated with later-life mental health problems including depressive-like behaviors and limbic system (amygdala and hippocampus) dysregulation.[57,58,61]

PEDIATRICS AND ATTACHMENT

Pediatric primary care provides a unique opportunity to detect infants at risk for attachment disorders.[76] Based on findings in basic research, specific observational tools have been developed for the use in primary care.[77] In a cross-sectional study of mothers and infants at an urban hospital clinic, the authors are currently assessing the prevalence of at-risk infants, using screening tools recommended by the American Academy of Pediatrics. Preliminary data analyses of 133 mother-infant dyads show that 34% of infants exhibit concerning behavior 6 months postpartum in this high-risk population of low socioeconomic status with a high prevalence of maternal psychiatric disorders (eg, 26% with maternal depression).[78] Finally, these findings underline the importance of translating results from basic research in human and animal studies into clinical practice and policy guidelines. Deciding how to make use of findings from basic research in pediatric practice, however, can be a challenging task. The newborns' preference for their mothers' smell, for example, has been successfully used to facilitate breastfeeding in both preterm and full-term babies.[79,80] There is likely no harm to mother or newborn in this practice, and the advantages of breastfeeding for both mother and newborn are well known.[81] Using the soothing effect of maternal odors to ease the newborn's discomfort 12 and pain[82] during invasive procedures, on the other hand, might not be an entirely judicious clinical decision, despite promising early results.[12] This practice might not only reduce the newborn's immediate stress response during the procedure but also reduce the clinician's stress response, because the newborn might cry less, as has been described in an excellent study by Goubet and colleagues.[82] Because odor conditioning has been demonstrated in newborns,[9] however, this practice could result in conditioning of the newborns who would learn to associate pain with their mother's odor. This is of particular importance for premature infants who undergo a multitude of painful procedures during their first months of life. In addition, premature infants often spend long periods separated from their mother; this might interfere with their ability to form a representation of their mother that integrates her odor with her warmth, voice, touch, and so forth. Associating maternal odor with pain might thus be confusing to the newborn and may interfere with development of bonding to the mother and secure attachment patterns. In summary, additional research is needed to clarify the role for maternal odor in clinical practice, following assessment of both short-term and long-term effects.[83]

CONCLUDING REMARKS

Infant attachment and bonding to the caregiver is widespread across animal species in which the survival of the young depends on a caregiver. The main function of attachment is to maintain contact between the infant and the caregiver to ensure infant survival. While infant-caregiver dyads are biologically predisposed to attach, learning about the caregiver is an additional determinant of the success and quality of attachment formation. The biological predisposition for attachment in infants seems to be mediated by a unique learning circuit that produces rapid, robust learning about the caregiver in both nurturing and abusive situations. Although attachment to an abusive caregiver seems contradictory, it may occur because the infant is programmed to ensure his or her own survival, which can only be achieved via continued contact with the caregiver, despite the poor quality of care provided. Attachment also contributes to infant developmental outcomes, such as emotionality, cognition, and overall mental health, as it is associated with specific caregiving patterns and levels of caregiving intensity. These specific patterns and intensity levels of stimulation to the infant's sensory systems can directly influence brain development.

Understanding this dual role of attachment in ensuring care and sculpting infant neural and behavioral development provides a unique perspective when determining the level of care required for premature infants. It remains difficult, however, to separate the effects of disrupted early-life attachment from the critical health issues associated with care of the preterm infant. Bidirectional translational research is key to advancing our understanding of attachment during the early infant period. Whereas human studies inform questions asked by animal researchers, animal research helps define mechanisms of basic functions and uncover unexpected results. Such interplay between human and animal research helps us optimize infant attachment formation, resulting in enhanced long-term outcomes for the both full-term and preterm infants.

REFERENCES

1. Bowlby J. John Bowlby and ethology: an annotated interview with Robert Hinde. Attach Hum Dev 2007;9(4):321–35.
2. Rutter M. Maternal deprivation reconsidered. J Psychosom Res 1972;16(4): 241–50.
3. DeCasper AJ, Fifer WP. Of human bonding: newborns prefer their mothers' voices. Science 1980;208(4448):1174–6.
4. Marlier L, Schaal B, Soussignan R. Neonatal responsiveness to the odor of amniotic and lacteal fluids: a test of perinatal chemosensory continuity. Child Dev 1998;69(3):611–23.
5. Moon CM, Fifer WP. Evidence of transnatal auditory learning. J Perinatol 2000; 20(8 Pt 2):S37–44.
6. Mennella JA, Johnson A, Beauchamp GK. Garlic ingestion by pregnant women alters the odor of amniotic fluid. Chem Senses 1995;20(2):207–9.
7. Schaal B, Marlier L, Soussignan R. Olfactory function in the human fetus: evidence from selective neonatal responsiveness to the odor of amniotic fluid. Behav Neurosci 1998;112(6):1438–49.
8. Fifer WP, Moon CM. The role of mother's voice in the organization of brain function in the newborn. Acta Paediatr Suppl 1994;397:86–93.
9. Sullivan RM, Taborsky-Barba S, Mendoza R, et al. Olfactory classical conditioning in neonates. Pediatrics 1991;87(4):511–8.
10. Fleming AS, O'Day DH, Kraemer GW. Neurobiology of mother-infant interactions: experience and central nervous system plasticity across development and generations. Neurosci Biobehav Rev 1999;23(5):673–85.
11. Varendi H, Porter RH. Breast odour as the only maternal stimulus elicits crawling towards the odour source. Acta Paediatr 2001;90(4):372–5.
12. Sullivan RM, Toubas P. Clinical usefulness of maternal odor in newborns: soothing and feeding preparatory responses. Biol Neonate 1998;74(6):402–8.
13. Rattaz C, Goubet N, Bullinger A. The calming effect of a familiar odor on full-term newborns. J Dev Behav Pediatr 2005;26(2):86–92.
14. Hofer M, Sullivan RM. Toward a neurobiology of attachment. In: Nelson C, Luciana M, editors. Handbook of developmental cognitive neuroscience. Cambridge (MA): MIT Press; 2001. p. 599–616.
15. Moon C, Bever TG, Fifer WP. Canonical and non-canonical syllable discrimination by two-day-old infants. J Child Lang 1992;19(1):1–17.
16. Schleidt M, Genzel C. The significance of mother's perfume for infants in the first weeks of their life. Ethol Sociobiol 1990;11(3):145–54.
17. Field TM, Cohen D, Garcia R, et al. Mother-stranger face discrimination by the newborn. Infant Behav Dev 1984;7(1):19–25.
18. Moon C, Cooper RP, Fifer WP. Two-day-olds prefer their native language. Infant Behav Dev 1993;16(4):495–500.
19. Marlier L, Schaal B, Soussignan R. Bottle-fed neonates prefer an odor experienced in utero to an odor experienced postnatally in the feeding context. Dev Psychobiol 1998;33(2):133–45.

20. Schaal B, Montagner H, Hertling E, et al. Olfactory stimulation in the relationship between child and mother. Reprod Nutr Dev 1980;20(3B):843–58 [in French].

21. Makin JW, Porter RH. Attractiveness of lactating females' breast odors to neonates. Child Dev 1989;60(4):803–10.

22. Valanne EH, Vuorenkoski V, Partanen TJ, et al. The ability of human mothers to identify the hunger cry signals of their own new-born infants during the lying-in period. Experientia 1967;23(9):768–9.

23. Kaitz M, Good A, Rokem AM, et al. Mothers' and fathers' recognition of their newborns' photographs during the postpartum period. J Dev Behav Pediatr 1988;9(4):223–6.

24. Cismaresco AS, Bonnin F. Evolution of maternal mood state and of the auditory and olfactory perception of their newborn: preliminary data. J Psychosom Obstet Gynaecol 1993;14(1):65–70.

25. Gustafson GE, Green JA, Cleland JW. Robustness of individual identity in the cries of human infants. Dev Psychobiol 1994;27(1):1–9.

26. Kaitz M, Lapidot P, Bronner R, et al. Parturient women can recognize their infants by touch. Dev Psychol 1992;28(1):35–9.

27. Porter RH. Olfaction and human kin recognition. Genetica 1998;104(3):259–63.

28. Blass EM, Teicher MH. Suckling. Science 1980;210(4465):15–22.

29. Mennella JA, Beauchamp GK. Maternal diet alters the sensory qualities of human milk and the nursling's behavior. Pediatrics 1991;88(4):737–44.

30. Balogh R, Porter R. Olfactory preference resulting from mere exposure in human neonates. Infant Behav Dev 1986;9:395–401.

31. Freud A. The infantile neurosis. Genetic and dynamic considerations. Psychoanal Study Child 1971;26:79–90.

32. Spitz RA. The psychogenic diseases in infancy—an attempt at their etiologic classification. Psychoanal Study Child 1951;6:255–75.

33. Robertson J. Young children in brief separation. A fresh look. Psychoanal Study Child 1971;26:264–315.

34. Lorenz K. The comparative method of studying innate behavioural patterns. Symp Soc Exp Biol 1950;4:221–68.

35. Mestzger M, Jiang S, Braun K. Organization of the dorsocaudal neostriatal complex: a retrograde and anterograde tracing study in the domestic chick with special emphasis on pathways relevant to imprinting. J Comp Neurol 1998;395(3):380–404.

36. Brock J, Schnabel R, Braun K. Role of the dorso-caudal neostriatum in filial imprinting of the domestic chick: a pharmacological and autoradiographical approach focused on the involvement of NMDA-receptors. Eur J Neurosci 2006;9(6):1262–72.

37. Harlow HF, Zimmermann RR. Affectional responses in the infant monkey; orphaned baby monkeys develop a strong and persistent attachment to inanimate surrogate mothers. Science 1959;130(3373):421–32.

38. Harlow HF, Suomi SJ. Social recovery by isolation-reared monkeys. Proc Natl Acad Sci U S A 1971;68(7):1534–8.

39. Weininger O, McClelland WJ, Arima RK. Gentling and weight gain in the albino rat. Can J Psychol 1954;8(3):147–51.

40. Levine S. Primary social relationships influence the development of the hypothalamic-pituitary-adrenal axis in the rat. Physiol Behav 2001;73(3):255–60.

41. Kleinhaus K, Steinfeld S, Balaban J, et al. Effects of excessive glucocorticoid receptor stimulation during early gestation on psychomotor and social behavior in the rat. Dev Psychobiol 2010;52(2):121–32.

42. Bowlby J. The making and breaking of affectional bonds. I. Aetiology and psychopathology in the light of attachment theory. An expanded version of the Fiftieth Maudsley Lecture, delivered before the Royal College of Psychiatrists, 19 November 1976. Br J Psychiatry 1977;130:201–10.

43. Ainsworth MD, Bell SM. Attachment, exploration, and separation: illustrated by the behavior of one-year-olds in a strange situation. Child Dev 1970;41(1):49–67.

44. Shannon C, Champoux M, Suomi SJ. Rearing condition and plasma cortisol in rhesus monkey infants. Am J Primatol 1998;46(4):311–21.

45. Hofer MA. Hidden regulators in attachment, separation, and loss. Monogr Soc Res Child Dev 1994;59(2-3):192–207.

46. Francis DD, Champagne FA, Liu D, et al. Maternal care, gene expression, and the development of individual differences in stress reactivity. Ann N Y Acad Sci 2006; 896:66–84.

47. Roth TL, Lubin F, Funk A, et al. Lasting epigenetic influence of early-life adversity on the BDNF gene. Biol Psychiatry 2009;65(9):760–9.

48. Bordner KA, Spear NE. Olfactory learning in the one-day old rat: reinforcing effects of isoproterenol. Neurobiol Learn Mem 2005;86(1):19–27.

49. Sullivan RM, McGaugh JL, Leon M. Norepinephrine-induced plasticity and one-trial olfactory learning in neonatal rats. Brain Res Dev Brain Res 1991;60(2): 219–28.

50. Raineki C, Pickenhagen A, Roth TL, et al. The neurobiology of infant maternal odor learning. Braz J Med Biol Res 2010;43(10):914–9.

51. Lagercrantz H, Slotkin TA. The "stress" of being born. Sci Am 1986;254:100–7.

52. Slotkin T, Seidler F. Adrenomedullary catecholamine release in the fetus and newborn: secretory mechanisms and their role in stress and survival. J Dev Physiol 1988;10(1):1–16.

53. Nelson EE, Panksepp J. Brain substrates of infant-mother attachment: contributions of opioids, oxytocin, and norepinephrine. Neurosci Biobehav Rev 1998; 22(3):437–52.

54. Hess EH. Imprinting and the critical period concept. In: Bliss EL, editor. Roots of behavior. New York: Hoeber-Harper; 1962. p. 254–63.

55. Salzen EA. Imprinting and environmental learning. In: Aronson LR, Tobach E, Lehrman DS, et al, editors. Development and evolution of behavior. San Francisco (CA): WH Freeman; 1970. p. 158–78.

56. Harlow HF, Harlow MK. The affectional systems. In: Schrier A, Harlow HF, Stollnitz F, editors. Behavior of nonhuman primates, vol. 2. New York: Academic Press; 1965. p. 287–344.

57. Roth T, Sullivan R. Memory of early maltreatment: neonatal behavioral and neural correlates of maternal maltreatment within the context of classical conditioning. Biol Psychiatry 2005;57(8):823–31.

58. Sullivan RM, Landers M, Yeaman B, et al. Good memories of bad events in infancy. Nature 2000;407(6800):38–9.

59. Hess E. Ethology: an approach to the complete analysis of behavior. In: Brown R, Galanter E, Hess E, et al, editors. New directions in psychology. New York: Holt, Rinehart and Winston; 1962. p. 159–99.

60. Stanley W. Differential human handling as reinforcing events and as treatments influencing later social behavior in basenji puppies. Psychol Rep 1962;10: 775–88.

61. Raineki C, Moriceau S, Sullivan RM. Developing a neurobehavioral animal model of infant attachment to an abusive caregiver. Biol Psychiatry 2010;67(12): 1137–45.

62. Maestripieri D, Tomaszycki M, Carroll KA. Consistency and change in the behavior of rhesus macaque abusive mothers with successive infants. Dev Psychobiol 1999;34(1):29–35.

63. Sanchez MM, Ladd CO, Plotsky PM. Early adverse experience as a developmental risk factor for later psychopathology: evidence from rodent and primate models. Dev Psychopathol 2001;13(3):419–49.

64. Fanselow M, Gale G. The amygdala, fear, and memory. Ann N Y Acad Sci 2003; 985:125–34.

65. LeDoux J. The emotional brain, fear, and the amygdala. Cell Mol Neurobiol 2003; 23:727–38.

66. Moriceau S, Wilson DA, Levine S, et al. Dual circuitry for odor-shock conditioning during infancy: corticosterone switches between fear and attraction via amygdala. J Neurosci 2006;26(25):6737–48.

67. Wiedenmayer CP, Barr GA. Developmental changes in c-fos expression to an age-specific social stressor in infant rats. Behav Brain Res 2001;126(1–2):147–57.

68. Davis M. Neurobiology of fear responses: the role of the amygdala. J Neuropsychiatry Clin Neurosci 1997;9:382–402.

69. Fanselow MS, LeDoux JE. Why we think plasticity underlying Pavlovian fear conditioning occurs in the basolateral amygdala. Neuron 1999;23(2):229–32.

70. Pape HC, Stork O. Genes and mechanisms in the amygdala involved in the formation of fear memory. Ann N Y Acad Sci 2003;985:92–105.

71. Rosenkranz JA, Grace AA. Dopamine-mediated modulation of odour-evoked amygdala potentials during pavlovian conditioning. Nature 2002;417(6886): 282–7.

72. Sigurdsson T, Doyere V, Cain CK, et al. Long-term potentiation in the amygdala: a cellular mechanism of fear learning and memory. Neuropharmacology 2007; 52(1):215–27.

73. Bauman MD, Lavenex P, Mason WA, et al. The development of mother-infant interactions after neonatal amygdala lesions in rhesus monkeys. J Neurosci 2004;24(3): 711–21.

74. Stone VE, Baron-Cohen S, Calder A, et al. Acquired theory of mind impairments in individuals with bilateral amygdala lesions. Neuropsychologia 2003;41(2): 209–20.

75. Tottenham N, Sheridan MA. A review of adversity, the amygdala and the hippocampus: a consideration of developmental timing. Front Hum Neurosci 2009;3:68.

76. Hagan JF Jr, Shaw JS, Duncan P. Bright futures guidelines for health supervision of infants, children, and adolescents. American Academy of Pediatrics; 2009.

77. Guedeney A, Fermanian J. The validity and reliability study of assessment and screening for sustained withdrawal reaction in infancy: the alarm distress baby scale. Infant Ment Health J 2001;22(5):559–75.

78. Burtchen N, Alvarez-Segura M, Dreyer BP, et al. Identifying infants at risk for social withdrawal behavior by utilizing the Edinburgh Postnatal Depression Screen (EPDS). International Society for Developmental Psychobiology Meeting. Washington, DC, November, 2011.

79. Raimbault C, Saliba E. The effect of the odour of mother's milk on breastfeeding behaviour of premature neonates. Acta Paediatr 2007;96(3):368–71.

80. Bingham PM, Churchill D, Ashikaga T. Breast milk odor via olfactometer for tube-fed, premature infants. Behav Res Methods 2007;39(3):630–4.

81. American Academy of Pediatrics. Breastfeeding and the use of human milk. In: American Academy of Pediatrics PS, editor. Pediatrics, vol. 115; 2005. p. 496–506.

82. Goubet N, Rattaz C, Pierrat V, et al. Olfactory experience mediates response to pain in preterm newborns. Dev Psychobiol 2003;42(2):171–80.
83. Liu WF, Laudert S, Perkins B, et al. The development of potentially better practices to support the neurodevelopment of infants in the NICU. J Perinatol 2007; 27:S48–74.

The Role of Early Auditory Development in Attachment and Communication

Christine Moon, PhD

KEYWORDS

- Critical period • Deafness • Language • Premature • Preterm
- Prenatal stimulation • Prenatal education

The sense of hearing begins to become functional during the second trimester of pregnancy. From that point on, the external world is available to the fetus in a way that is immediate, rich, and faithful to the original stimulus. This stimulation is unlike other sensory signals except for slower vibrations through the maternal body that vary in frequency and intensity in real time. Reliable fetal movement in response to loud external sound has been measured as early as 27 weeks of pregnancy,[1] which means that development is nearing the point of the full sensory experience of signal detection, perception (including attention and recognition), and action. Because human life is social, fetal auditory experience is characterized by sounds of social activity, especially voices. The maternal voice dominates but other voices are available.[2,3] This means that social behavior such as attachment and communication may be established before birth through auditory experience. Infants and children flourish when they have enduring social and emotional bonds, and when they communicate well. Thus, it is important to understand how social behavior develops along with how the brain organizes itself using available sensory input, in this case auditory signals. This article presents research results from the study of audition as it emerges during the perinatal period for typically developing individuals, and it focuses on incipient attachment and communication systems as served by audition. The article discusses attachment and communication in cases of atypical auditory experience such as sound deprivation in deafness or the experience of developmentally unexpected

Financial disclosure/conflicts of interest: the author has nothing to disclose.
Funding provided by National Institutes of Health Grant HD 37954 to Patricia K. Kuhl, University of Washington, Seattle, USA.
Department of Psychology, Pacific Lutheran University, 12180 Park Avenue South, Tacoma, WA 98447, USA
E-mail address: mooncm@plu.edu

Clin Perinatol 38 (2011) 657–669
doi:10.1016/j.clp.2011.08.009
0095-5108/11/$ – see front matter © 2011 Elsevier Inc. All rights reserved.

sound as in prolonged hospitalization of preterm newborns. The practice of providing extra auditory stimulation to the fetus is discussed, and the article questions the function of very early auditory experience for good attachment and communication outcomes.

FETAL AUDITION

After decades of research with fetuses of different species, including humans, and with newborn preterm infants, it is clear that humans are capable of hearing a variety of sounds for about 3 months before birth. For a thorough recent review of fetal and neonatal auditory development, see Granier-Deferre and colleagues.[4]

The cochlea is functional by around 24 weeks' gestational age (GA),[5] and an ultrasound study showed that, by 27 weeks, 96% of fetuses responded with movement to loud (up to 120 dB) pure tones of 100 to 500 Hz.[1] Fetal magnetoencephalography (fMEG) has revealed auditory discrimination of loud pure tones (120 dB) in the brains of some individuals as early as 28 weeks' GA.[6] This is remarkable because it represents activity in the auditory cortex even while cochlear biomechanics are still developing, eventually becoming mature at 35 weeks.[7] The auditory cortex continues to mature in the weeks leading up to birth and continues to develop through the first years of life.[8] As the auditory system develops through the last weeks of gestation, the fetus becomes progressively more responsive to high-pitched tones,[1] which is consistent with the development of response along the basilar membrane of the cochlea from low to high frequencies.[9] Detection thresholds and response latencies both decline with time as the auditory system matures.[1,6]

In addition to the research showing detection of pure tones, studies with late-term fetuses and neonates show that they are capable of perceiving and acting on aspects of sound that play a role in attachment and communication during the first year of postnatal life. Research strategies include measuring fetal and newborn discrimination of familiar versus unfamiliar sounds as well as measuring newborn preference for familiar sounds. Studies have shown differential responding by the fetus to the maternal voice compared with an unfamiliar voice[10,11] (although not all researchers have found this[12]) or a story recited by the mother compared with a novel story.[13,14] Neonates with less than 2 hours' postnatal experience respond selectively to the maternal voice with more motor activity compared with the sound of an unfamiliar voice.[15] Newborns less than 3 days of age alter their sucking patterns to activate a recording of the maternal voice, indicating that the voice can act as a reinforcer.[16–18] Similarly, a recording of heartbeats acts as a reinforcer for change in sucking behavior.[19] In an fMEG study measuring brain activity to the maternal heartbeat, in contrast with externally generated pure tones, late-term fetuses showed a response that did not habituate over time. The investigators explained the failure to habituate as being caused by the inherent variability in rhythm and loudness of the maternal heartbeat.[20] Learning experiments using controlled prenatal exposure to music have shown that neonates respond to a familiar melody on postnatal days 3 to 5,[21,22] and at 1 month of postnatal age.[23] The retention of musical sound is consistent with the idea that the musical qualities of voice (pitch, loudness and rhythm) are salient in the perinatal experience of speech.[2,22,24] Newborns selectively respond to speech samples carrying information about whether the speaker is happy or not,[25] information that is based on pitch, loudness, and rhythm. However, the fetus is not limited to these slower-changing speech characteristics but rather is also capable of detecting[26,27] and discriminating[28,29] much briefer speech sounds, namely the vowel sounds ah or ee. These vowels are different from each other in acoustics and articulation, and they were good candidates for discrimination. By 38 weeks' GA, the fetus is capable of processing acoustic streams with variations in sound spectra and amplitude over short and long time intervals with a transient orienting heart rate response to music and a sustained response to speech.[4] During the neonatal period, infant-controlled laboratory procedures show that infants prefer to hear speech compared with a similar nonspeech stimulus,[30] and they differentiate the maternal native language from a foreign language.[31] They prefer to hear the maternal language rather than a foreign language,[32] and newborns of bilingual women show an equivalent response for both of their mother's languages.[33] In a remarkable demonstration of precocity, newborns match the pitch contours of their cries to the predominant contour of their native language.[34] Thus, a growing body of research shows that, at the time of their birth, infants have already experienced and mentally processed a rich auditory world including aspects of sound that will come to signal the presence of particular individuals in their lives as well as the those acoustic signals that communicate mental states and linguistic messages.

DEVELOPMENT OF ATTACHMENT

The emotional attachment of the infant to his or her mother has potential precursors in the intrauterine experience of sounds associated with mother, such as her talking, her laughter, her songs, and her heartbeats. Intrauterine recordings show that the maternal voice has a privileged status among voice sounds, if not in clarity, then in intensity,[3,35] total amount of exposure, and likely in a route that has sensory redundancy. Each occurrence of maternal voicing is accompanied by perfectly timed motion that is matched in intensity to the intensity of the auditory signal. When mother is speaking, singing, laughing, or coughing, she is likely to also be causing motion that is available to her fetus from her diaphragm, her gestures, and other body actions. In perinatal experiments with another species that is attuned at birth to the maternal auditory signal (quail), concurrent auditory and vestibular stimulation provides redundant information from two different senses and has been shown to enhance subsequent attention to the maternal call.[36] If this is the case for humans, sensory redundancy is a contributor to the salience of mother's voice at birth.

Within hours and days after birth, newborn infants alter their behavior to activate recordings of the maternal voice, her language, familiar music, familiar stories, and heartbeats. This preferential behavior on the part of neonates is proximity-seeking according to attachment theory as originally proposed by John Bowlby,[37] a British psychiatrist. Informed by an ethological approach that emphasizes innate species-typical predispositions, Bowlby[37] was influenced by his observations of institutionalized infants and children who had failed to make emotional attachments during early development. Experiments by Harlow and Harlow[38] with infant rhesus monkeys showed that infant proximity-seeking with a comfort figure is not unique to humans and that failure to attach is detrimental to development. Human infants form emotional attachments with caregivers other than the mother, but Bowlby[37] and subsequent researchers described a primary attachment figure who is most often the baby's mother. Regarding their study of neonatal preference for the maternal voice, DeCasper and Fifer[16] stated that "mother-infant bonding would best be served by (and may even require) the ability of a newborn to discriminate its mother's voice from that of other females."[16(p1174)]

Proximity-seeking characterizes all developmental phases of the attachment process and, in the case of a newborn, include the use of "the infant's perceptual equipment and the way it tends to orient him toward his mother-figure" and "his effector equipment, notably hands and feet, head and mouth, which, when given a chance, tend to latch him in contact with her."[37(p271)] In proximity-seeking, the sense of hearing is advantaged compared with other senses because it allows contact at a distance when the mother is unavailable through touch, smell, or sight. With its early maturation and the advantage of audition in caregiver contact, it is plausible that this sensory system plays an important role in the development of attachment.

LANGUAGE DEVELOPMENT

If the early development of audition is likely to play a key role in socioemotional attachment, it most certainly plays one in communication for most people. The major mode of human communication is language, and, for all but a minority of people, language is oral/aural. There are indications that most elements of the speech signal are available to the fetus, at least intermittently. Intrauterine audio recordings made during labor after rupture of membranes in humans[35] and in fetal lamb cochlea[39] show that speech prosody (pitch variation, rhythm, and stress) is faithfully represented and that even the phonemes (vowels and consonants) are intelligible in about 30% of the recorded words and syllables. The available spectral composition and temporal variation are sufficient to allow the fetus to generate different attentional responses to speech versus music,[4] to discriminate between 2 vowels,[28,29] and even to learn the acoustic patterns in a familiar story.[13,14] As parents, clinicians, and researchers know, immediately following birth and thereafter, infants are attentive to voices. Babies bring their prenatal experience with speech into their postnatal life, including a preference for a story read out loud prenatally by mother[32,40] and for the maternal language.[32] The familiar story and language preferences were expressed in studies using unfamiliar voices, showing that the newborns had learned speaker-general characteristics of the speech signal. Researchers have suggested that fetal and perinatal attentiveness to, and memory for, vocal language, particularly the prosodic aspects of speech, may launch infants into reading caregiver emotions[25] and also into language acquisition.[4,22,24,41]

SENSITIVE PERIODS

A notable aspect of both attachment and language acquisition is that they are experience-dependent and that there are sensitive or critical periods for both. As studies of institutionalized children have shown, early isolation increases the risk of subsequent poor attachment and mental health despite a later opportunity to form an emotional bond with a caregiver.[42] Similarly, children who have not been exposed to speech by early childhood are not likely to acquire completely normal use of spoken language.[43,44] Recent evidence that indicates the parameters of a sensitive period for language acquisition comes from studies of prelingually deaf children who receive cochlear implants (CIs) at varying ages and therefore go from being deaf to hearing.[45]

Sensitive or critical periods for language and attachment are caused by the early neural plasticity that is necessary for experience to sculpt the brain's architecture and inform the developing neurochemistry that serves emotional development[46] and language.[47] After the period of plasticity ends, the experiences of having a sensitive caregiver or hearing spoken language do not result in recovery from deprivation. Because auditory contributors to attachment and speech perception seem to be present during the fetal and newborn periods, and because the sensitive periods end early in life, an important question is whether fetal and perinatal auditory experience of a certain kind is necessary for the development of spoken language or for socioemotional attachment. A potential answer for this question lies in cases in which prenatal auditory stimulation has been deviant: excessive, absent or impoverished, or different from what is normally provided by the environment.

EXCESSIVE SOUND

Excessive noise damages the auditory system, particularly the hair cells of the cochlea, but little research has been done on the effect of prenatal exposure to excessive noise. Controlled exposure of fetal sheep to loud noise increased postnatal auditory brainstem response thresholds, and resulted in damage to cochlear hair cells.[48] In humans, retrospective studies have shown that women who experienced loud occupational noise while pregnant had children with increased risk for hearing loss.[49,50] Thus it is clear that prenatal exposure to excessive high-intensity sound interferes with the auditory system's ability to detect sound; however, the doses and timing relationships are not known. It is also not known whether or how much excessive prenatal sound exposure damages auditory processing beyond the cochlea, independent of damage to the cochlea itself. Moreover, there is an alternate pathway by which excessive sound may disrupt the developing auditory system, and that is through maternal stress. When pregnant rats were exposed to mild stressors (handling, novel cages, saline injections) the pups subsequently had increased auditory brainstem response thresholds for detecting low-frequency tones.[51] Excessive noise is a human stressor,[52] and, if the results from rats are reliable,[53] and if they extend to humans, it is possible that noise-induced stress during pregnancy affects auditory system development, and that the effects are not limited to the peripheral auditory system.

DEAFNESS

Many other factors besides excessive prenatal noise can compromise the early development of the auditory system. Approximately 2 to 3 in 1000 infants are born deaf or hard of hearing, 90% of whom are born to parents who can hear.[54] Infants who have little or no prenatal or early postnatal exposure to auditory stimulation are test cases for the importance of audition to the development of attachment and communication, especially spoken language. The research literature on deafness and language acquisition is plentiful, but the literature on deafness and attachment is lacking. For reviews and recommendations on deafness and early attachment, see Refs.[55,56] Studies of attachment are typically conducted beginning at 1 year of age using the Strange Situation,[57] a procedure originally devised by Mary Ainsworth, who had worked with John Bowlby. The Strange Situation procedure has been widely adopted as a valid measure of the infant and toddler's emotional connection to the primary caregiver. In the procedure, the toddler enters into conflict between exploring toys and remaining close to the caregiver in the presence of unfamiliar setting and people. According to attachment theory, an individual baby's behavior reflects the internal working model of the caregiver as a more or less dependable source for meeting the baby's needs.[58]

For children younger than 1 year, a measure of the mother-infant relationship is the face-to-face interaction. Typically there is synchrony between the looking behavior of the infant and the caregiver. The infant makes a bid for mother's attention by gazing intently at mother's face. The social interaction ensues. During the interaction, the infant breaks gaze to dampen overarousal and self-regulate emotional intensity. Ideally, the mother responds to her baby's initial bid for attention and also allows the infant to self-regulate by not intruding on the gaze aversion.[59]

Research indicates that there are some differences in face-to-face interaction among mother-infant dyads who differ in their hearing status. For example, deaf infants, regardless of whether their mothers are deaf or hearing, look away less often, perhaps because they rely heavily on visual contact. In deaf mother–deaf infant interactions, after the infant's bid for attention, the mother delivers exaggerated facial expressions, gestures, and signs; the equivalent of motherese speech. Hearing mothers of deaf infants are less likely to use these nonverbal cues. Another difference is that, during the deaf infant's attempt to self-regulate by gaze aversion, the hearing mother is likely to take action to bring her infant back into interaction. Overall, in their conclusions regarding a longitudinal study of 4 groups of mother-infant dyads who were either alike or opposite in their hearing status, Meadow-Orlans and colleagues[55] concluded that "it must be emphasized that although many differences existed among the four groups of mothers and infants, there were even more similarities in their behaviors."[(p55)] This indicates that emotional attachment of deaf infants can proceed successfully without auditory input.

For older deaf infants and toddlers, there is similarly little rigorous research on attachment, with only 1 investigation that included all 4 types of mother-infant hearing status dyads using the well-studied Strange Situation test.[55] In that study, deaf 18-month-olds did not differ from hearing infants in the numbers who were rated as securely attached, the category with the best attachment outcome. However, there was a higher proportion of deaf than hearing infants who were classified as avoidant, meaning that they did not seek proximity to get relief from distress on reunion with mother after a brief separation. Attachment theory says that a history of not being able to use the caregiver as a secure base results in avoidant behavior, but there are cultural differences. The deaf toddlers' increased avoidant status mirrors that of German children who may have mothers who culturally parent for early independence. The investigators question whether the Strange Situation is well-suited to measuring attachment in deaf children because (1) the toddlers are accustomed to mother leaving without a prominent signal such as a door closing, or (2) mothers of deaf children may adopt parenting practices that encourage a lack of dependence on others.[55] The investigators' conclusion is that difficulties with attachment in deaf infants can be attributed to the child's ecological system, not to a lack of auditory input.[55,56]

Compared with studies of infant attachment, there is more research on language acquisition by infants who have no auditory experience including the acquisition of manual as well as spoken language. Therefore, there is abundant information about the contribution of early auditory experience to oral/aural communication. Because a minority of deaf individuals use oral language, deaf mothers who have hearing infants present an interesting case because their infants are not exposed to much prenatal and early postnatal maternal speech. Despite the lack of early exposure to spoken language, the children meet major milestones on time in 2 languages: sign and spoken language. They receive sufficient exposure to spoken language from non-maternal sources to become proficient, often serving as interpreters at an early age for their deaf parent(s).[55] This finding suggests that, although the typical fetal experience includes learning about spoken language from the mother's voice, it is not necessary for language acquisition.

The recent practice of extending CI surgery to prelingually deaf infants and toddlers has created a natural experiment on the critical/sensitive period for acquisition of spoken language. Implantation at various ages and subsequent tests of different types of receptive and expressive language skills provide data about the timing of sensitive periods for all levels of spoken language use from phonetics to grammar. Investigators of a recent review of implantation of cochlear devices at different ages concluded that "Taken together, the data from AEPs (auditory evoked potentials), functional imaging studies, animal models, and audiologic outcomes indicate that there appears to be a sensitive period – though perhaps not a true critical period – for implantation that goes beyond the simple notion that earlier is better. At some point, between the ages of 2 and 4 years, the plasticity of the auditory system begins to decline sharply; thereafter the benefits of cochlear implantation are greatly reduced."[45(p246)] Research on hearing children of deaf mothers and on prelingually deaf CI recipients bears directly on the question of the necessity of fetal and newborn auditory experience for oral/aural language acquisition. Results suggest that there is sufficient plasticity in the developing auditory system for normal spoken language acquisition in the absence of the rich prenatal and early postnatal auditory experience that is available for the developing infant.

HOSPITALIZED PRETERM INFANTS

Hospitalized preterm infants have neither excessive nor impoverished auditory experience during early development, but their experience is markedly different from what is typical for late-term gestation. These infants' early development occurs in medical settings in which guidelines regarding excessive sound have been implemented, and sound levels are controlled.[60,61] Even in environments in which loud, percussive sound has been eliminated, the spectral and temporal composition of sound is not the same as what would have been available to the developing auditory system in the womb. In general, sound in utero is characterized by progressive attenuation of frequencies of more than 500 Hz, with some exceptions caused by the resonance characteristics of the intrauterine environment.[3,35,62] Thus, preterm infants are exposed to higher frequencies at greater intensities compared with fetuses of comparable GA. Moreover, they do not experience the sensory redundancy of speech and motion.

Although infants and children born before term have been shown to have increased incidence of sensorineural hearing loss,[63] auditory neuropathy spectrum disorder,[64] and language development problems,[65] it is unclear whether unusual auditory input during the perinatal period plays a role. If the cause of hearing loss associated with prematurity is multifactorial,[66] then the cause of language deficits involves even more factors because general cognitive abilities are necessary in addition to auditory-specific ones.[67] For children with normal hearing, early brain anomalies as well as later postdischarge environmental conditions have emerged as predictors of language skills at 5 years of age.[68,69] These factors do not implicate abnormal auditory experience. However, it is possible that the aberrant sound environment affects later language acquisition in subtle ways that have yet to be understood. An example might be a deficit in rapid auditory processing abilities (RAP). RAP is a response to auditory events that occur in quick succession, on the order of milliseconds, as in speech perception. A deficit in RAP in infancy is related to poorer language outcomes in toddlers and preschoolers.[70] A training program with rapidly occurring auditory events seems to ameliorate the condition in older children.[71] A recent longitudinal magneto-encephalography study on fetal and full-term newborn brain responses to 2 brief, successive tones revealed a response that was not present during the fetal period but gradually developed in the first 3 postnatal weeks, with evidence of successful processing by 22 days. The investigators concluded that RAP develops in the first 3 weeks after term birth and that further investigation will reveal the roles of experience with speech sounds and brain maturation.[72] Although it is a speculative proposal,[73] these results suggest a way that the aberrant auditory experience of preterm infants may affect later language processing. They also suggest a pathway to very early intervention for a particular deficit. Whether the auditory experience of hospitalized preterm infants has an enduring effect on the development of RAP is unknown, but it provides an example of a subtle influence on the ability to communicate in the absence of overt hearing loss.

FUNCTION OF PRENATAL AUDITORY EXPERIENCE AND PLASTICITY

The evidence reviewed earlier shows that the late-term fetus typically has had abundant experience with sounds of the social environment, and that important bases for attachment and language are present at birth. There also is evidence that individuals without such bases at birth nevertheless establish healthy attachments with caregivers and acquire spoken language. It is reasonable to ask what functions fetal auditory perception and learning serve if not preparation for vital postnatal functions like attachment and spoken language. It may be that prenatal auditory experience functions primarily to develop the well-practiced ability to detect and to perceive a salient sound and to act on the perception.[74] For most infants, perception and action entail recognized sounds, but there are infants who, beginning shortly after birth, never hear the same prenatal voices or language again. Their brains are adaptively prepared to attend to and rapidly learn to recognize the new voices and speech sounds. Plasticity also serves those individuals who experienced little or no sound at all until their second or third year, as well as those who were born early and did not get the full time with species-typical prenatal sounds. The cortex is apparently open to organization by speech sound stimulation until between 3 and 4 years of age, depending on the task.[45] It is not known whether the later-organized cortex is the same as in children who have been hearing since before birth. This is an exciting area for both basic and applied research.

FETAL STIMULATION PROGRAMS

If late-term fetuses are able to detect, perceive, and take action (eg, by directing their attention) when stimulated with sound, then the question arises as to whether it is possible or desirable to educate the unborn child. It is clear that it is possible. The late-term fetus retains the experience of a melody for up to a month after birth.[23] Is it desirable? From the perspective of the parents' or siblings' attachment to the infant who will shortly arrive, it could be part of a healthy transition to a changed family. Mother's voice is available each time she speaks, so no extra maternal stimulation seems necessary. However, it may help siblings or father to get close to the pregnant belly and talk or sing to the new family member. Music from the radio, television, or stereo is available to the fetus,[75] as presumably are environmental sounds such as the vacuum cleaner, the dog barking, or car door slamming shut.

Some people have advocated going further with prenatal education than simply talking normally to the fetus. There are commercially available fetal stimulation programs that advise the use of small audio speakers that are strapped directly onto the maternal belly. Despite claims to the contrary, there is no evidence that this practice is beneficial, and there is potential harm from too much stimulation. Although many sound frequencies are attenuated in the womb, low frequencies and some higher ones are naturally unattenuated and may even be amplified,[2,3,62] so, if some frequencies are amplified by the belly device to be sufficiently loud, the unattenuated ones may be very loud. Moreover, an important advance during late gestation is increasing differentiation and regulation of sleep-wake states. Recurrent noise has been shown to adversely affect sleep/wake states in preterm infants[76] and in term infants,[77] and it may affect sleep/wake states in the fetus. On the grounds that there is no evidence of benefit to stimulation from audio speakers in contact with the pregnant belly, and there is reason to be concerned about overstimulation, it is at best a questionable practice and at worst a harmful one.

SUMMARY

Several conclusions can be drawn from studies of perinatal auditory development. There is no doubt that auditory perception and learning take place for most typically developing fetuses. Sounds of social life are prominent in the intrauterine environment, and they provide opportunities for prenatal learning about eventual attachment figures and language(s). Typical development includes prenatal learning about ambient social sounds, but fetuses and newborns who lack the typical auditory exposure nonetheless can go on to develop typical socioemotional attachment and the ability to communicate well, as measured by experimental methods. Processes for acquisition of spoken language have sufficient plasticity to recover from early deprivation until 3 to 4 years of age if good support is provided. Hospitalized preterm infants experience sounds that deviate from those that are expected by the developing auditory system. It is not known whether any subsequent hearing and language-processing deficits are caused solely by early deviant auditory experience or by other medical and/or family resource factors. Plasticity through the first 3 years, shown in cases of sound deprivation, suggests that detrimental effects of deviant early exposure to sounds may be remediated by later experience.

Although experience and learning take place in the womb, it is not the case that more is better. Prenatal stimulation in the form of amplified sound from audio speakers in contact with the maternal belly is not advisable because of the potential for excessive exposure to sound that may disrupt development of the auditory system and sleep/wake state organization.

REFERENCES

1. Hepper PG, Shahidullah BS. Development of fetal hearing. Arch Dis Child 1994; 71(2):F81–7.
2. Querleu D, Renard X, Boutteville C, et al. Hearing by the human fetus? Semin Perinatol 1989;13(5):409–20.
3. Richards DS, Frentzen B, Gerhardt KJ, et al. Sound levels in the human uterus. Obstet Gynecol 1992;80(2):186–90.
4. Granier-Deferre C, Ribeiro A, Jacquet AY, et al. Near-term fetuses process temporal features of speech. Dev Sci 2011;14(2):336–52.
5. Pujol R, Laville-Rebillard M, Lenoir M. Development of sensory and neural structures in the mammalian cochlea. In: Rubel EW, Popper AN, Fay RR, editors. Development of the auditory system. Springer handbook of auditory research. New York: Springer-Verlag; 1998. p. 146–93.
6. Draganova R, Eswaran H, Murphy P, et al. Serial magnetoencephalographic study of fetal and newborn auditory discriminative evoked responses. Early Hum Dev 2007;83(3):199–207.
7. Morlet T, Collet L, Salle B, et al. Functional maturation of cochlear active mechanisms and of the medial olivocochlear system in humans. Acta Otolaryngol 1993; 113(3):271–7.
8. Moore JK, Guan YL. Cytoarchitectural and axonal maturation in human auditory cortex. J Assoc Res Otolaryngol 2001;2(4):297–311.
9. Gray L, Rubel EW. Development of absolute thresholds in chickens. J Acoust Soc Am 1985;77(3):1162–72.

10. Kisilevsky BS, Hains SM, Lee K, et al. Effects of experience on fetal voice recognition. Psychol Sci 2003;14(3):220–4.
11. Smith LS, Dmochowski PA, Muir DW, et al. Estimated cardiac vagal tone predicts fetal responses to mother's and stranger's voices. Dev Psychobiol 2007;49(5): 543–7.
12. Hepper PG, Scott D, Shahidullah S. Newborn and fetal response to maternal voice. J Reprod Infant Psychol 1993;11(3):147–53.
13. DeCasper AJ, Lecanuet JP, Busnel MC, et al. Fetal reactions to recurrent maternal speech. Infant Behav Dev 1994;17(2):159–64.
14. Krueger C, Holditch-Davis D, Quint S, et al. Recurring auditory experience in the 28- to 34-week-old fetus. Infant Behav Dev 2004;27(4):537–43.
15. Querleu D, Lefebvre C, Titran M, et al. Reactivite du nouveau-ne de moins de deux heures de vie a la voix maternelle. J Gynecol Obstet Biol Reprod (Paris) 1984;13:125–35 [in French].
16. DeCasper AJ, Fifer WP. Of human bonding: newborns prefer their mothers' voices. Science 1980;208(4448):1174–6.
17. Fifer WP, Moon CM. Early voice discrimination. In: von Euler C, Forssberg H, Lagercrantz H, editors. Neurobiology of early infant behaviour. New York: Stockton Press; 1989. p. 277–86.
18. Moon CM, Bever TG, Fifer WP. Canonical and non-canonical syllable discrimination by two-day-old infants. J Child Lang 1992;19:1–17.
19. DeCasper AJ, Sigafoos AD. The intrauterine heartbeat: a potent reinforcer for newborns. Infant Behav Dev 1983;6:19–25.
20. Porcaro C, Zappasodi F, Barbati G, et al. Fetal auditory responses to external sounds and mother's heart beat: detection improved by independent component analysis. Brain Res 2006;1101(1):51–8.
21. James DK, Spencer CJ, Stepsis BW. Fetal learning: a prospective randomized controlled study. Ultrasound Obstet Gynecol 2002;20:431–8.
22. Panneton Cooper R, Aslin RN. The language environment of the young infant: implications for early perceptual development. Can J Psychol 1989;43(2): 247–65.
23. Granier-Deferre C, Bassereau S, Ribeiro AL, et al. A melodic contour repeatedly experienced by human near-term fetuses elicits a profound cardiac reaction one month after birth. PLoS One 2011;6(2):e17304.
24. Nazzi T, Bertoncini A, Mehler J. Language discrimination by newborns: toward an understanding of the role of rhythm. J Exp Psychol Hum Percept Perform 1998; 24(3):756–66.
25. Mastropieri DP, Turkewitz G. Prenatal experience and neonatal responsiveness to vocal expressions of emotion. Dev Psychobiol 1999;35(3):204–14.
26. Zimmer EZ, Fifer WP, Kim Y, et al. Response of the premature fetus to stimulation by speech sounds. Early Hum Dev 1993;33:207–15.
27. Groome LJ, Mooney DM, Holland SB, et al. Temporal pattern and spectral complexity as stimulus parameters for eliciting a cardiac orienting reflex in human fetuses. Percept Psychophys 2000;62(2):313–20.
28. Lecanuet J, Granier-Deferre C, DeCasper AJ, et al. Perception et discrimination foetales de stimuli langagiers; mise en evidence a partir de la reactivite cardiaque; resultats preliminaires. C R Acad Sci III 1987;305(3):161–4 [in French].
29. Shahidullah S, Hepper PG. Frequency discrimination by the fetus. Early Hum Dev 1994;36(1):13–26.
30. Vouloumanos A, Werker JF. Listening to language at birth: evidence for a bias for speech in neonates. Dev Sci 2007;10(2):159–64.

31. Bertoncini J, Bijeljac-Babic R, Jusczyk PW, et al. An investigation of young infants' perceptual representations of speech sounds. J Exp Psychol Gen 1988;117(1):21–33.
32. Moon C, Panneton Cooper R, Fifer WP. Two-day-olds prefer their native language. Infant Behav Dev 1993;16(4):495–500.
33. Byers-Heinlein K, Burns TC, Werker JF. The roots of bilingualism in newborns. Psychol Sci 2010;21(3):343–8.
34. Mampe B, Friederici AD, Christophe A, et al. Newborns' cry melody is shaped by their native language. Curr Biol 2009;19:1–4.
35. Querleu D, Renard X, Versyp F, et al. Fetal hearing. J Gynecol Obstet Biol Reprod 1988;28(3):191–212.
36. Lickliter R, Bahrick LE, Markham RG. Intersensory redundancy educates selective attention in bobwhite quail embryos. Dev Sci 2006;9(6):604–15.
37. Bowlby J. Attachment and loss: vol. 1. Attachment. New York: Basic Books; 1969.
38. Harlow HF, Harlow M. Social deprivation in monkeys. Sci Am 1962;207:136–46.
39. Smith SL, Gerhardt KJ, Griffiths SK, et al. Intelligibility of sentences recorded from the uterus of a pregnant ewe and from the fetal inner ear. Audiol Neurootol 2003; 8(6):347–53.
40. DeCasper AJ, Spence MJ. Prenatal maternal speech influences newborns' perception of speech sounds. Infant Behav Dev 1986;9:133–50.
41. Moon CM, Fifer WP. Evidence of transnatal auditory learning. J Perinatol 2000; 20(8):S37–44.
42. Bos K, Zeanah CH, Fox NA, et al. Psychiatric outcomes in young children with a history of institutionalization. Harv Rev Psychiatry 2010;19(1):15–24.
43. Fromkin V, Krashen S, Curtiss S, et al. The development of language in genie: a case of language acquisition beyond the 'critical period'. Brain Lang 1974; 1(1):81–107.
44. Mayberry RI, Lock E. Age constraints on first versus second language acquisition: evidence for linguistic plasticity and epigenesis. Brain Lang 2003;87(3): 369–84.
45. Peterson NR, Pisoni DB, Miyamoto RT. Cochlear implants and spoken language processing abilities: review and assessment of the literature. Restor Neurol Neurosci 2010;28(2):237–50.
46. Weaver IC, Cervoni N, Champagne FA, et al. Epigenetic programming by maternal behavior. Nat Neurosci 2004;7(8):847–54.
47. Kuhl PK, Conboy BT, Padden D, et al. Early speech perception and later language development: implications for the 'critical period'. Lang Learn Dev 2005;1(3–4):237–64.
48. Gerhardt KJ, Pierson LL, Huang X, et al. Effects of intense noise exposure on fetal sheep auditory brain stem response and inner ear histology. Ear Hear 1999;20(1): 21–32.
49. Daniel T, Laciak J. Observations cliniques et experiences concernant l'etat de l'appareil cochleovestibulaire des sujets exposes au bruit durant la vie foetale. Rev Laryngol Otol Rhinol (Bord) 1982;103:313–8 [in French].
50. Lalande NM, Hetu R, Lambert J. Is occupational noise exposure during pregnancy a high risk factor of damage to the auditory system of the fetus? Am J Ind Med 1986;10:427–35.
51. Kadner A, Pressimone VJ, Lally BE, et al. Low-frequency hearing loss in prenatally stressed rats. Neuroreport 2006;17(6):635–8.
52. Szalma JL, Hancock PA. Noise effects on human performance: a meta-analytic synthesis. Psychol Bull 2011;137(4):682–707.

53. Hougaard KS, Barrenas ML, Kristiansen GB, et al. No evidence for enhanced noise induced hearing loss after prenatal stress or dexamethasone. Neurotoxicol Teratol 2007;29(6):613–21.

54. National Institute on Deafness and Other Communication Disorders. Statistics about hearing, balance, ear infections and deafness. Available at: http://www.nidcd.nih.gov/health/statistics/Pages/quick.aspx. Accessed September 30, 2011.

55. Meadow-Orlans KP, Spencer PE, Koester LS. The world of deaf infants: a longitudinal study. New York: Oxford University Press; 2004.

56. Thomson NR, Kennedy EA, Kuebli JE. Attachment formation between deaf infants and their primary caregivers: is being deaf a risk factor for insecure attachment? In: Zand DH, Pierce KJ, editors. Resilience in deaf children: adaptation through emerging adulthood. New York: Springer Science+Business Media; 2011. p. 27–64.

57. Ainsworth MD, Bell SM. Attachment, exploration, and separation: illustrated by the behavior of one-year-olds in a strange situation. Child Dev 1970;41(1):49–67.

58. Bretherton I, Gunnar MR, Sroufe LA. Pouring new wine into old bottles: the social self as internal working model. In: Gunnar MR, Sroufe LA, editors. Self processes and development. Hillsdale (NJ): Lawrence Erlbaum Associates; 1991. p. 1–41.

59. Beebe B. Co-constructing mother-infant distress in face-to-face interactions: contributions of microanalysis. Zero Three 2004;24(5):40–8.

60. Graven SN. Sound and the developing infant in the NICU: conclusions and recommendations for care. J Perinatol 2000;20:S88–93.

61. Philbin MK, Robertson A, Hall JW 3rd. Recommended permissible noise criteria for occupied, newly constructed or renovated hospital nurseries. The Sound Study Group of the National Resource Center. J Perinatol 1999;19(8 Pt 1):559–63.

62. Lecanuet JP, Gautheron B, Locatelli A, et al. What sounds reach fetuses: biological and nonbiological modeling of the transmission of pure tones. Dev Psychobiol 1998;33(3):203–19.

63. Hille ET, van Straaten HI, Verkerk PH. Prevalence and independent risk factors for hearing loss in NICU infants. Acta Paediatr 2007;96(8):1155–8.

64. Coenraad S, Goedegebure A, van Goudoever JB, et al. Risk factors for auditory neuropathy spectrum disorder in NICU infants compared to normal-hearing NICU controls. Laryngoscope 2011;121(4):852–5.

65. Wolke D, Samara M, Bracewell M, et al. Specific language difficulties and school achievement in children born at 25 weeks of gestation or less. J Pediatr 2008;152(2):256–62.

66. Coenraad S, Goedegebure A, van Goudoever JB, et al. Risk factors for sensorineural hearing loss in NICU infants compared to normal hearing NICU controls. Int J Pediatr Otorhinolaryngol 2010;74(9):999–1002.

67. Wolke D. Language problems in neonatal at risk children: towards an understanding of developmental mechanisms. Acta Paediatr 1999;88(5):488–90.

68. Inder TE, Warfield SK, Wang H, et al. Abnormal cerebral structure is present at term in premature infants. Pediatrics 2005;115(2):286–94.

69. Hopkins-Golightly T, Raz S, Sander CJ. Influence of slight to moderate risk for birth hypoxia on acquisition of cognitive and language function in the preterm infant: a cross-sectional comparison with preterm-birth controls. Neuropsychology 2003;17(1):3–13.

70. Benasich AA, Tallal P. Infant discrimination of rapid auditory cues predicts later language impairment. Behav Brain Res 2002;136(1):31–49.

71. Gaab N, Gabrieli JD, Deutsch GK, et al. Neural correlates of rapid auditory processing are disrupted in children with developmental dyslexia and ameliorated with training: an fMRI study. Restor Neurol Neurosci 2007;25(3–4):295–310.

72. Sheridan CJ, Matuz T, Draganova R, et al. Fetal magnetoencephalography - achievements and challenges in the study of prenatal and early postnatal brain responses: a review. Infant Child Dev 2010;19(1):80–93.

73. Ortiz-Mantilla S, Choudhury N, Leevers H, et al. Understanding language and cognitive deficits in very low birth weight children. Dev Psychobiol 2008;50(2): 107–26.

74. Lecanuet JP, Granier-Deferre C, DeCasper A, et al. Are we expecting too much from prenatal sensory experiences? In: Hopkins B, Johnson SP, editors. Prenatal development of postnatal functions. Westport (CT): Praeger Publishers; 2005. p. 31–49.

75. Hepper PG. Fetal "soap" addiction. Lancet 1988;1(8598):1347–8.

76. Wachman EM, Lahav A. The effects of noise on preterm infants in the NICU. Arch Dis Child Fetal Neonatal Ed 2011;96(4):F305–9.

77. Ando Y, Hattori H. Effects of noise on sleep of babies. J Acoust Soc Am 1977; 62(1):199–204.

Early Visual Development: Implications for the Neonatal Intensive Care Unit and Care

Stanley N. Graven, MD

KEYWORDS

• Premature infant • Endogenous stimuli • Visual development
• NICU • Melanopsin • Epigenetics • Human

Much of the early development of the human visual system occurs while the preterm infant is in the neonatal intensive care unit (NICU). Critical events and processes occur between 20 and 40 weeks' gestational age, before the onset of vision at term birth. Knowledge of the development of the visual system and the timing of the processes involved is essential to adapting NICU care to support all neurosensory development including visual development.

The human visual system is the most thoroughly studied of the sensory systems. Studies from the 1950s and 1960s created the framework for much of the subsequent research. It was the work of Hubel and Wiesel[1,2] in the 1960s on the need for and role of visual experience that became the basis for much of the research through the 1970s and 1980s. Shatz and coworkers[3,4] continued with the studies of retinal function and the development of the retinogeniculate pathway. LeVay and colleagues[5] continued the work on the development of ocular dominance columns in the visual cortex and the effects of visual deprivation. New technology for studying the brain has greatly advanced the studies of the human visual system.

The sensory systems of humans and other mammals develop sequentially in clearly defined periods or stages. The main sensory systems with critical developmental periods in late fetal and neonatal life are listed in **Table 1**. The visual system is the last to develop functionally. Protecting the development of the visual system remains important because visual problems continue to be common among NICU graduates who were preterm births.

Department of Community and Family Health, College of Public Health, University of South Florida, 13201 Bruce B. Downs Boulevard, MDC 56, Tampa, FL 33612-3805, USA
E-mail address: sgraven@health.usf.edu

Clin Perinatol 38 (2011) 671–683
doi:10.1016/j.clp.2011.08.006
0095-5108/11/$ – see front matter © 2011 Elsevier Inc. All rights reserved.

Table 1
Neurosensory systems with early critical periods

1. Limbic system	Emotion and feeling
2. Hippocampus	Memory, early sensory development, brain plasticity
3. Chemosensory	
a. Olfactory	Smell
b. Gustatory	Taste
4. Somatosensory	Touch, pressure, vibration, temperature, pain
5. Kinesthetic proprioception: vestibular	Position and movement Balance and motion
6. Auditory	Hearing
7. Visual	Vision

THE COMPONENTS OF THE VISUAL SYSTEM
The Eye, Eyelids, and Optics

The cornea, iris, lens, and eyelids are all parts of the optic function (**Fig. 1**). The eyelids and iris control the amount of light entering the eye, whereas the lens provides focus and image detail. Infants at or before 32 weeks' gestation have thin eyelids and little or no pupillary constriction. This allows little ability to limit light reaching the retina.[5] By 34 to 36 weeks' gestation, the pupillary constriction is more consistent and the eyelids are thicker, allowing some ability to limit light exposure to the retina. There is no developed pathway for an image to reach the visual cortex in utero and the fetus in utero has no exposure to light or visual image. The pathways from the retina to the visual cortex that transmit visual images become functional at 39 to 40 weeks' gestation. Preterm birth does not accelerate the maturation of the human visual system, although it

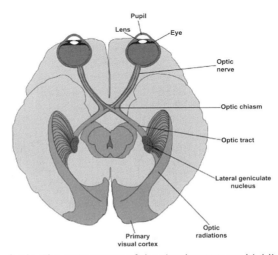

Fig. 1. The human brain. The components of the visual system are highlighted and labeled. (*Data from* Hubel DH. Eye, brain, and vision. New York: Scientific American Library; 1988.)

does introduce a need for some light exposure to entrain the circadian rhythm that was maintained by the mother in utero.[6-9]

The Retina

The cellular components of the retina and their connections are shown in **Fig. 2**. Cones are formed early and concentrate centrally. As the retina grows, the rods develop and migrate to the periphery where they are less dense.[10,11] The location of the rods and cones determines the distribution of the other retinal cellular elements.

There are 3 layers of cells and 2 synaptic layers or regions (see **Fig. 2**). The photoreceptor cells differ according to type of photopigment. The bipolar, amocrine, and retinal ganglion cells (RGCs) differ primarily by the presence of either glycine or glutamate receptors resulting in On or Off signal neurons. This provides forward and feedback signals which modulate the intensity of the visual image.[8,12-14] The On or Off characteristics that relate to the glycine or glutamate receptors reverse their function with the onset of vision at term. The timing of this reversal is not altered or accelerated by preterm birth. Müller glial cells are structural elements that provide the genetic signal molecules which direct the axon and dendrite growth from the RGCs.[15]

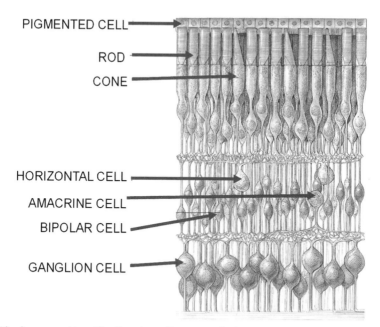

Fig. 2. The human retina. The 5 major cell types and 3 layers are shown. Not shown are the Müller glial cells, which are structural and extend across the thickness of the retina from the ganglion cell layer to the pigmented layer, or the center-surround photoreceptor system. The relationship of the horizontal and amacrine cells to the photoreceptor is essential to the operation of the center-surround system for visual reception. (*From* Hubel DH. Eye, brain and vision. New York: Scientific American Library; 1988; with permission. A cross section of the retina, about midway between the fovea and far periphery, where rods are more numerous than cones. From top to bottom is about one-quarter millimeter.)

The outer layer of the retina is composed of photoreceptor cells that are activated by light or images. This layer is composed of rods and cones, which are the 2 major groups of photoreceptors. The rods and cones connect to bipolar cells. Between the photoreceptor layer and the bipolar cells are horizontal cells that form a synaptic network linking rods and cones to groups of bipolar cells. The bipolar cells connect to the RGCs. Some bipolar cell connections go directly to ganglion cells and some connect though amocrine cells. This part of the internal regulatory system of the retina processes the visual signals that are transmitted to the ganglion cells and ultimately to the visual cortex.[8,11] The RGC axons connect to the lateral geniculate nucleus (LGN) (see **Fig. 1**).

The cells of the human and mammalian retina arise from cell division and differentiation. From research on the ferret, the timing of their appearance is shown in **Fig. 3**.[16] The bipolar cells are the last to develop and are not needed until after the ganglion cells, rods, cones, and horizontal and amocrine cells have been formed. In utero, this all occurs in the absence of light or exogenous visual stimulation. Extrauterine visual experience in preterm primates and humans can produce synaptic overproduction and alterations in the visual system cells and connections.[17,18]

LGN

The LGN cells begin development at 10 to 12 weeks' gestation. The RGC axons synapse with the LGN cells beginning at 15 weeks. The LGN cell axons create synapses with the visual cortex beginning at 25 weeks' gestation. The LGN is composed of 6 layers. Lamina or layers begin to form at 22 weeks and continue to term at 40 weeks. The RGCs have synapses throughout the LGN by term, and this creates the topographic relationship between the retina and the LGN, as well as between the LGN and the visual cortex.[19]

Superior Colliculus

The superior colliculus (SC) is the target for some of the RGC axons. The SC begins development early in gestation and begins receiving afferent axons from the RGCs

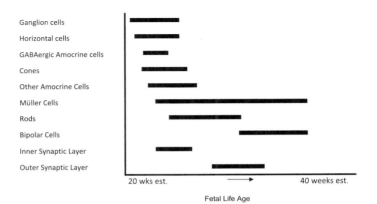

Fig. 3. Timing of retinal cell appearance. (*Data from* Lamb TD, Collin SP, Pugh EN Jr. Evolution of the vertebrate eye: opsins, photoreceptors, retina and eye cup. Nat Rev Neurosci 2007;8(12):960–76.)

around 15 weeks. Afferents from the SC create synapses in areas related to ocular movement and gaze regulation. The afferents from the visual cortex also connect with the SC. These connections are essential for the development of eye movement, gaze control, and binocular vision.[19] A portion of the SC is responsible for integrating visual, auditory, and touch stimuli related to perception of shape and space in 3 dimensions.

Visual Cortex

The visual cortex is located in the occipital lobe of the brain. It is composed of 6 layers of cells that originate in the germinal matrix and migrate to the occipital cortex early in gestation. These cells are stimulated by endogenous waves of activity from the RGC to move into vertical columns with lateral connections. These columns are the ocular dominance columns and the orientation columns, which are created before birth. These columns are cell alignments that prepare the visual cortex for exogenous visual experience.

All of the processes involved in the development of the structure and function of the human visual system described earlier have a critical period between 20 and 40 weeks' gestation during which epigenetic events, toxic exposures, and inappropriate exogenous stimulation can produce significant alterations in the structure and function of the infant's visual system.

HUMAN VISUAL SYSTEMS

Human vision is composed of 3 subsystems that develop sequentially and have distinct functions at different stages of development. The 3 subsystems are (1) the melanopsin nonimage light-only system; (2) the scotopic, rod-based system, which functions at low light levels and transmits light and images but not color; and (3) the photopic system, which operates at higher light levels and transmits images, motion, and color.

The Melanopsin System

The melanopsin system is the most recently described. For many years, investigators observed that blind animals still respond physiologically to light and dark. This response to light and dark was seen when rods and cones were eliminated or blocked but the eyes remained. This response was lost when the eyes were physically removed. Provencio and colleagues[20] established that this system was based on cells containing a photopigment that he named melanopsin. He also discovered photoactive melanopsin-containing RGCs in mammals that responded directly to light without connections to rods, cones, or bipolar cells, now called intrinsically photosensitive retinal ganglion cells (ipRGC).[21] The melanopsin pigment and melanopsin-containing cells have peak activation by light of a wavelength around 480 nm and function between 459 and 484 nm in the turquoise-blue spectrum. This function differs from the 3 primary pigments in the cones that are responsible for color vision.[22] The ipRGC are only 1% or less of all RGCs at birth and decrease in number in early neonatal life. They are activated directly by light or receive stimuli from melanopsin-containing rods and cones via bipolar cells. None of the axons of the ipRGC connect to the visual cortex.

The ipRGC axons innervate or connect to many nuclei and brain regions, the most important of which are listed in **Table 2**.[23] These ipRGC axons transmit light-only stimuli that activate the areas noted. They are important for many functions that are coordinated with visual image stimuli later in development. For an excellent review

Table 2
Brain regions innervated by ipRGCs with their general functions

ipRGC Target	Function
1. Suprachiasmatic nucleus	Regulation of circadian rhythms
2. Intergeniculate leaflet	Integration of photic and nonphotic circadian cues
3. Olivary thalamic nucleus	Pupillary constriction
4. Posterior thalamic nucleus	Nociception: painful or injurious stimuli Processing of thalamic, cortical, and visual signals
5. SC	Integration of modalities for gaze control
6. LGN	Image-forming vision; visual motor function
7. Ventrolateral preoptic nucleus	Promotion of sleep

Data from Do MT, Yau KW. Intrinsically photosensitive retinal ganglion cells. Physiol Rev 2010;90(4):1547–81.

of the ipRGC and function see Do and colleagues.[23] The melanopsin system is responsible for circadian photoentrainment, pupillary light reflex, sleep regulation, and suppression of pineal melatonin production. The ipRGC axons also connect to the LGN and SC for integration of the modalities needed for gaze control and visual motor functions, but do not transmit image, motion, or color to the visual cortex. These functions appear later as the scotopic and photopic subsystems develop. The melanopsin system requires more light than the rod-based scotopic system and less light than the cone-based photopic system. The melanopsin ipRGC system and its multiple brain connections develop in utero with endogenous stimulation, but in the absence of light. However, with preterm birth, the ipRGC respond to light in the melanopsin wavelength range and activate certain brain connections. This response occurs in the absence of the functional bipolar cells, which are necessary for transmission of light, image, motion, and color from the retina to the visual cortex. As the melanopsin system matures, it develops melanopsin-containing rods and cones that then connect to the ipRGC via bipolar cells; this occurs at or near term. Alterations in the development of connections which result from premature light exposure are reflected in problems of gaze control and binocular coordination, which are common in NICU graduates who were born preterm. Most of these problems appear later as the scotopic and photopic systems develop. Stimulation of the ipRGC can occur in the preterm infant and can affect entrainment of the circadian clock and, perhaps, other related functions that would have been provided in utero The melanopsin system continues to develop and integrate into the function of the scotopic and photopic systems during the early months of neonatal life. The melanopsin system is essential throughout life and is responsible for many neurophysiologic functions unrelated to vision.

The Scotopic System

The scotopic system is based on the rod photoreceptors, which function at very low light (VLL) levels. It develops during the later weeks of fetal life and becomes functional at birth near term.[9] The function of the scotopic system begins with the maturation of the rod bipolar cells. It is the primary system for image vision in the early months of neonatal life.

There are 4 basic types of rods. Two types function at VLL levels. Multiple VLL rods connect to a single VLL rod bipolar cell that connects to a single RGC. This allows weak signals from VLL stimuli to be summated and thus creating a stronger signal to the LGN and visual cortex. The third type of rod operates at a higher light level and connects to a cone bipolar cell for connection to a ganglion cell. This provides for greater detail for the image. These rods are activated by light of a wide range of wavelengths but do not have the specific photopigments of cones that are needed to distinguish color. The fourth type, the melanopsin-containing rods, connects to the melanopsin bipolar cells and the ipRGC as part of the melanopsin system. With growth of the eye during development, the rods concentrate in the periphery of the retina, which is why peripheral vision is used in low light conditions (ie, night vision).

The Photopic Visual System

The photopic visual system is based on the cone visual receptors. They are formed early in the photoreceptor layer and are primarily located centrally in the retina. This system provides the center focus for vision.

The human retina has 3 types of cones based on the visual pigments and their light sensitivity.[24] These 3 types of cones are each maximally sensitive to light of specific ranges of wavelengths. The blue cones have activation peaks at 424 nm, the green cones transmit at a peak of 530 nm, and the orange-red cones peak at 560 nm. The brain cannot perceive color from a single cone, but must receive signals from 2 or more separate cone types to compare wavelengths.[24] The cones are the receptors that transmit images and color, but require higher levels of light. The cones connect to 1 or more of several types of bipolar cells. The bipolar cells either connect directly to RGCs or connect via an amocrine cell (see **Fig. 2**).[5] These connections form the photopic visual system. The cone receptors become active after the rod receptors and thus the photopic visual system develops after the rod-based scotopic system. The photopic system is not fully functional for color or image until 3 to 4 months of neonatal life.

The horizontal cells are slow potential cells that remain polarized as long as there is stimulation. This process is needed to sustain an image. These cells modulate photoreceptor signals as well as feedback signals. There are 2 physiologic types of horizontal cells. The C-type horizontal cell connects cones to groups of bipolar cells that are needed for image and color, and the L-type horizontal cell functions to balance signals of differing levels of luminosity. Horizontal cells are in the outer synaptic layer (see **Fig. 2**) and are essential for the center-surround visual response system.[8] They become functional after 40 weeks' gestation.

The amocrine cells are part of the inner synaptic layer. These cells are essential for the synchronous waves of RGC activation that are needed for the topographic alignment of cells in the LGN and columns in the visual cortex. They also provide feedback to the rod bipolar cells and other functions associated with the low light (scotopic) vision.[8,11] Later-developing amocrine cells are associated with the center-surround visual system in conjunction with horizontal cells. The center-surround visual system is needed to create a sharp image and detail.[25] It becomes functional around 5 to 6 months of age. Attention and an image that is in focus are essential for the early visual experience of infants.

From the retina, the RGC axons connect to the LGN, which is the primary relay area from the eye to the visual cortex. As the LGN matures, the cells migrate into 6 layers that match the topographic arrangement of the retina. The neurons from the LGN connect to the visual cortex. The development of cell columns with lateral connections in the visual cortex is essential for a functional photopic visual system.

Processes Involved in Visual Development

There are 3 primary or basic processes involved in early brain development that apply specifically to neurosensory development. This article focuses on their role in visual development. These processes are:

1. Genetic and epigenetic processes
2. Endogenous brain activity
3. Exogenous neurosensory stimulation.

Genetics and Epigenetics

The earliest processes of visual development are genetically coded and involve cell division, differentiation, and migration, and the structure of the neurosensory systems. These processes all occur without specific outside or endogenous stimulation. For many years, genetics (DNA) was considered to be solely responsible for the structure of the visual system.

The discovery of epigenetic processes in the past 20 or more years has altered the understanding of the role of genetics in neurodevelopment. Epigenetics involves the alteration in gene expression by environmental, neuroendocrine, neurophysiologic, and other events or exposures that can alter gene expression without altering the basic gene DNA.

It is now evident that synaptic connections and cell alignments can be significantly altered by epigenetic processes resulting from changes in maternal or fetal physiology or adverse factors in the environment. In DNA, between the active genes are inactive DNA segments as well as structures called histones. The maternal fetal environment, NICU and infant care environment, toxic exposures, severe and prolonged stress, and the constant exposure to catecholamines are all factors that can alter the expression of the genes without changing the basic DNA. The processes involved are methylation of the DNA, histone methylation, phosphorylation or acetylation, and/or the creation of noncoding microRNAs, which are the epigenetic mechanisms that are responsible for the changes in gene expression. They not only can affect the mother and fetus but can alter germ cells of the fetus and thus pass the alterations on to the next generation; a transgenerational effect.[26] Epigenetic alteration that occurs during fetal and early prenatal life can be expressed at any time into adult life.[27–30]

Endogenous Brain Activity

The initial location of neuroganglion cells and other neural cells may occur as a result of genetic or epigenetic signals, but they need stimulation to move to their functional location and connect with the appropriate targets. For the visual system development, there is a critical period during which cell realignment can occur, but only with the appropriate endogenous stimulation.

Endogenous stimulation is created by spontaneous firing of neural cells, mostly ganglion cells, which occurs at a particular time in their development. The spontaneous endogenous neural cell activities occur in the retina, LGN, SC, hippocampus, pons, cerebellum, cerebral cortex, spinal cord, and auditory systems. These locations all generate endogenous cell stimulation.[31–36]

The knowledge of endogenous stimulation and its timing is essential for caregivers, because it occurs during the last 12 to 14 weeks of fetal life and the early months of neonatal life. Some endogenous stimulation needs to occur over a lifetime. For the visual system, the RGCs are the first to fire. They begin as random firing and progress to regular firing, which is needed to stimulate the growth and targeting of the RGC axons with cells in the LGN and SC and create the topographic alignment.

The maturation of starburst amocrine cell occurs between 24 and 29 weeks gestation. The cells are required for the synchronous waves of firing of the RGCs. The synchronous waves alternate between eyes and are essential for the topographical organization of the LGN and the development of ocular dominance and orientation columns in the visual cortex.[32,37,38] Ocular dominance columns and orientation columns are needed for creation and selection of directional columns when the infant's eyes are open after birth at term.

At 29 to 30 weeks' gestation, the sleep partitions into rapid eye movement (REM) and non-REM (slow-wave) sleep. The sleep patterns are initially discontinuous with brief sleep patterns interspersed with periods of minimally organized electrical activity.[39–41]

By 32 to 34 weeks, RGC waves are coordinated with pontine-geniculato-occipital (PGO) waves from the pons in the brain stem and θ waves from the hippocampus in the temporal lobe as sleep cycles mature. The synchronous RGC waves, the PGO waves from the pons, and the θ waves from the hippocampus only occur during REM sleep. The transition to regular sleep cycles occurs around 30 to 34 weeks' gestation.[41] Any event, process, or drug that disrupts REM sleep or blocks the RGC waves and PGO waves from the pons will disrupt the organization of the LGN, visual cortex, and other visual system connections. Protecting sleep cycles, and especially REM sleep periods, is critical for healthy visual development.

Exogenous Stimulation

The endogenous stimulation of the visual system prepares the retina, LGN, and visual cortex for exogenous or outside stimulation. The human visual system at 40 weeks' gestation has intact retinal development and pathways to the visual cortex. At that time, the visual system must have regular visual stimulation. At 40 weeks, the infant can distinguish lines, patterns, movement, and differing light intensities, but not color. The rod-based scotopic visual system provides the vision until 2 to 3 months of age when the photopic system begins to add color and detail. Red is the first color the infant discriminates.

The ocular dominance and orientation columns developed in utero form the framework and connections for the selection of directional columns that result from external visual stimuli. Directional columns are required for seeing lines, patterns, and movement. They develop between birth at 40 weeks and 7 to 8 months of age. There must be columns in the visual cortex for lines, shapes, and movement in all directions. Separate columns are needed to see lines for each 5° of arc, which are essential to recognize all parts of a visual image or pattern.[42] These directional columns fail to develop if the infant is deprived of specific exogenous visual experiences. Columns for depth perception and complex pattern perception and comparison develop during the first 3 years of life. The visual cortex and the visual columns continue to make connections to the temporal lobe, parietal lobe, prefrontal cortex, and nuclei associated with gaze and eye movement through the early years of childhood.

Visual experience for healthy visual development requires (1) ambient light (not direct light); (2) focus; (3) attention; (4) novelty; (5) movement; and, after 2 to 3 months, (6) color.[41]

VISUAL DEVELOPMENT: IMPLICATIONS FOR CARE IN THE NICU ENVIRONMENT

The limbic system (emotions), olfactory system (smell), somatosensory system (touch), kinesthetic proprioceptive system (movement), and auditory systems all respond to external stimuli by 25 to 28 weeks' gestation and exhibit in utero learning. Developmentally appropriate care practices are designed to respond to the developmental needs of each of these systems. The visual system is not developmentally ready for external visual stimuli until birth at term. The visual system develops in utero in the total absence of light or image stimulation. Care practices for the preterm infant are designed to protect the endogenous processes needed for visual development as well as preventing interference with the development of the other sensory systems.

There are 3 main areas of care in the NICU that can adversely affect visual development in the preterm infant. These are:

1. Interference with endogenous brain cell activity.
   The synchronous firing of the RGC, the P wave from the pons, the θ waves from the hippocampus, and the firing of the cells that are part of the melanopsin system are all essential for healthy visual development.
2. Sleep deprivation.
   The endogenous waves of brain activity require sleep cycles, and especially REM sleep. Disruption in REM sleep in experimental animals consistently results in significant alterations in visual development.
3. Intense light exposure.
   Intense light exposure activates photoreceptors before the development of bipolar cells and thus no signals go to the RGCs or the pathways to the visual cortex. This omission can create abnormalities in the retinal organization and immature visual system. It can also create interference with the development of other sensory systems, especially the auditory system.[43]

Preterm Infants, Very Low Birth Weight, 22 to 28 Weeks Gestation

For the visual system during this period, the important care issues are protection of the eyes from direct light and keeping ambient light exposure to low levels. It is also important to limit exposure to drugs that can depress the endogenous firing of the cells involved in the early visual development.

The Intermediate Preterm Infant, 28 to 36 Weeks' Gestation

Between 28 and 36 weeks, the endogenous stimulation from the RGC, especially the synchronous waves of ganglion cells firing in the retina and LGN, begins the orderly creation of the topographic relationship between the retina, LGN, and visual cortex where the ocular dominance and orientation columns are forming. This period is also the time when the melanopsin visual system completes many connections to the nonimage areas of the visual system (see **Table 2**).

During this period, the PGO waves from the pons are added to the synchronous waves from the RGCs, leading to the creation of the ocular dominance and orientation columns and developing connections to the other parts of the cerebral cortex in preparation for scotopic vision at 39 to 40 weeks' gestation. During this time, intense atypical stimulation (noise, vibration, disturbing stimuli) of the other sensory systems can interfere with the processes of visual system development.[43] The impact is both direct interference with neuroprocesses and indirect interference with sleep cycles, especially REM sleep. REM sleep is essential for the organization of the intraretinal connections, the topographic alignment, and the development of the ocular dominance and orientation columns in the visual cortex.

In the NICU, it is important to have care that supports the development of the sensory systems that precede vision in the developmental sequence. For the visual system during this period, the developmental care needs are:

1. Protect the eyes from direct light exposure and maintain low levels of ambient light when not needed for care and procedures.
2. Provide some daily exposure to light, preferably including the shorter wavelengths, for entrainment of the circadian rhythm.
3. Protect sleep cycles, and especially REM sleep. Avoid sleep interruptions, bright lights, loud noises, and unnecessary physical disturbing activities.
4. Avoid high doses of sedative and depressing drugs, which can interfere with RGC waves, PGO waves, and hippocampal θ waves. These waves are all are essential for the visual system development.
5. Provide developmental care appropriate for the age and maturation of the infant.

The Late Preterm Infant, 36 to 39 Weeks' Gestation

During this period, the melanopsin (ipRGC) visual system should be well developed with the primary connection complete (see **Table 2**). The scotopic, rod-based visual system should be completed with the maturation of the rod bipolar cells near term, which provides for transmission of both image and light, but not color, to the visual cortex. After 40 weeks, the cortex requires visual experience in humans for development of directional columns, and thus needs active outside visual stimuli.[44]

State Organization

The preterm infant does not need vision for state organization before term. Most attempts by parents and caregivers to create visual engagement or interaction only disturb the sleep cycles and endogenous brain activity. The preterm infant begins state organization in response to warmth, skin-to-skin touch, voice and auditory stimulation, chemosensory stimuli, and gentle motion. Short periods of visual exposure to light in the melanopsin wavelength range is the only visual stimulation of value. Excessive and early exposure to intense or flickering light can alter the synaptogenesis in the visual system as well as the auditory system.[17,25,43] This can alter the expected development of these systems.

Once infants reach the age of 39 to 40 weeks, they need interactive visual experiences. The social and emotional context and atmosphere matter as much as the visual experience. Parents of preterm infants who graduate from the NICU need to understand the type and content of the interaction required for continued development in the early months of postterm life. The problems observed in the follow-up of infants who were preterm and in the NICU are related both to events associated with the NICU environment and to the environment and care received after discharge. All preterm infants require long-term follow-up of visual function for early detection of visual problems, which are common in preterm NICU graduates.

REFERENCES

1. Hubel DH, Wiesel TN. Receptive fields, binocular interaction and functional architecture in the cat's visual cortex. J Physiol 1962;160:106–54.
2. Hubel DH, Wiesel TN. The period of susceptibility to the physiological effects of unilateral eye closure in kittens. J Physiol 1970;206(2):419–36.
3. Shatz CJ, Kirkwood PA. Prenatal development of functional connections in the cat's retinogeniculate pathway. J Neurosci 1984;4(5):1378–97.

4. Shatz CJ, Stryker MP. Prenatal tetrodotoxin infusion blocks segregation of retino-geniculate afferents. Science 1988;242(4875):87–9.

5. LeVay S, Wiesel TN, Hubel DH. The development of ocular dominance columns in normal and visually deprived monkeys. J Comp Neurol 1980;191(1):1–51.

6. Fenichel GM. The neurological consultation. Neonatal neurology. 2nd edition. New York: Churchill Livingstone; 1985. p. 1–23.

7. Fielder AR, Foreman N, Moseley MJ, et al. Prematurity and visual development. Early visual development: normal and abnormal. New York: Oxford University Press; 1993. p. 485–504.

8. Kolb H. How the retina works - much of the construction of an image takes place in the retina itself through the use of specialized neural circuits. Am Sci 2003; 91(1):28–35.

9. Reeves A. Visual adaptation. In: Chalupa LM, Werner JS, editors. The visual neurosciences. Cambridge (MA); London: MIT; 2004. p. 851–62.

10. Swaiman KF. Neurologic examination of the preterm infant. In: Swaiman KF, editor. Pediatric neurology: principles and practice. St Louis (MO): Mosby; 1994. p. 61–72.

11. Wong RO, Godinho L. Development of the vertebrate retina. In: Chalupa LM, Werner JS, editors. The visual neurosciences. Cambridge (MA): MIT Press; 2004. p. 77–93.

12. Chiu C, Weliky M. The role of neural activity in the development of orientation selectivity. In: Chalupa LM, Werner JS, editors. The visual neurosciences. Cambridge (MA): MIT Press; 2004. p. 117–25.

13. Marquardt T, Gruss P. Generating neuronal diversity in the retina: one for nearly all. Trends Neurosci 2002;25(1):32–8.

14. Maslim J, Webster M, Stone J. Stages in the structural differentiation of retinal ganglion cells. J Comp Neurol 1986;254(3):382–402.

15. Reichenbach A, Pannicke T. Neuroscience. A new glance at glia. Science 2008; 322(5902):693–4.

16. Lamb TD, Collin SP, Pugh EN Jr. Evolution of the vertebrate eye: opsins, photo-receptors, retina and eye cup. Nat Rev Neurosci 2007;8(12):960–76.

17. Bourgeois JP, Jastreboff PJ, Rakic P. Synaptogenesis in visual cortex of normal and preterm monkeys: evidence for intrinsic regulation of synaptic overproduc-tion. Proc Natl Acad Sci U S A 1989;86(11):4297–301.

18. Tsuneishi S, Casaer P. Effects of preterm extrauterine visual experience on the development of the human visual system: a flash VEP study. Dev Med Child Neurol 2000;42(10):663–8.

19. Boothe RG. Visual development: central neural aspects. In: Meisami E, Timiras PS, editors. Handbook of human growth and developmental biology, Neural, sensory, motor and integrative development. Pt B: Sensory, motor, and integrative development, vol. 1. Boca Raton (FL): CRC Press; 1988. p. 179–91.

20. Provencio I, Jiang G, De Grip WJ, et al. Melanopsin: an opsin in melanophores, brain, and eye. Proc Natl Acad Sci U S A 1998;95(1):340–5.

21. Provencio I. The hidden organ in your eyes. Sci Am 2011;304(5):54–9.

22. Brainard GC, Sliney D, Hanifin JP, et al. Sensitivity of the human circadian system to short-wavelength (420-nm) light. J Biol Rhythms 2008;23(5):379–86.

23. Do MT, Yau KW. Intrinsically photosensitive retinal ganglion cells. Physiol Rev 2010;90(4):1547–81.

24. Goldsmith TH. What birds see. Sci Am 2006;295(1):68–75.

25. Graven SN. Early neurosensory visual development of the fetus and newborn. Clin Perinatol 2004;31(2):199–216.

26. Lubin FD. Epigenetic gene regulation in the adult mammalian brain: multiple roles in memory formation. Neurobiol Learn Mem 2011;96(1):68–78.
27. Nelson ED, Monteggia LM. Epigenetics in the mature mammalian brain: effects on behavior and synaptic transmission. Neurobiol Learn Mem 2011;96(1):53–60.
28. Nelissen EC, van Montfoort AP, Dumoulin JC, et al. Epigenetics and the placenta. Hum Reprod Update 2011;17(3):397–417.
29. Nugent BM, McCarthy MM. Epigenetic underpinnings of developmental sex differences in the brain. Neuroendocrinology 2011;93(3):150–8.
30. McKay JA, Mathers JC. Diet induced epigenetic changes and their implications for health. Acta Physiol (Oxf) 2011;202(2):103–18.
31. Goodman CS, Shatz CJ. Developmental mechanisms that generate precise patterns of neuronal connectivity. Cell 1993;72(Suppl):77–98.
32. Feller MB. Spontaneous correlated activity in developing neural circuits. Neuron 1999;22(4):653–6.
33. Penn AA, Shatz CJ. Brain waves and brain wiring: the role of endogenous and sensory-driven neural activity in development. Pediatr Res 1999;45(4 Pt 1): 447–58.
34. Penn AA, Shatz CJ, Lagercrantz H, et al. Principles of endogenous and sensory activity-dependent brain development. The visual system. The newborn brain: neuroscience and clinical applications. Cambridge (MA); New York: Cambridge University Press; 2002. p. 204–225.
35. Penn AA, Riquelme PA, Feller MB, et al. Competition in retinogeniculate patterning driven by spontaneous activity. Science 1998;279(5359):2108–12.
36. Penn AA. Early brain wiring: activity-dependent processes. Schizophr Bull 2001; 27(3):337–47.
37. Wong RO, Meister M, Shatz CJ. Transient period of correlated bursting activity during development of the mammalian retina. Neuron 1993;11(5):923–38.
38. Meister M, Wong RO, Baylor DA, et al. Synchronous bursts of action potentials in ganglion cells of the developing mammalian retina. Science 1991;252(5008): 939–43.
39. Fielder AR, Moseley MJ, Ng YK. The immature visual system and premature birth. Br Med Bull 1988;44(4):1093–118.
40. Graven SN, Browne JV. Visual development in the human fetus, infant, and young child. Newborn Infant Nurs Rev 2008;8(4):194–201.
41. Graven S. Sleep and brain development. Clin Perinatol 2006;33(3):693–706.
42. Hubel DH. Eye, brain and vision. New York: Scientific American Library; 1988.
43. Lickliter R. The role of sensory stimulation in perinatal development: insights from comparative research for care of the high-risk infant. J Dev Behav Pediatr 2000; 21(6):437–47.
44. Chapman B, Godecke I, Bonhoeffer T. Development of orientation preference in the mammalian visual cortex. J Neurobiol 1999;41(1):18–24.

The Prefrontal-Limbic System: Development, Neuroanatomy, Function, and Implications for Socioemotional Development

Katharina Braun, PhD

KEYWORDS

- Brain development • Emotion • Learning • Memory
- Amygdala • Hippocampus • Prenatal stress • Neonatal stress

DEFINITION, ANATOMY, AND FUNCTIONS

The neurologist Paul Broca[1] coined the term "limbic lobe" (*limbic* is derived from the Latin word *limbus*, which means *circle*) for several brain regions located underneath the cortex that form a ring around the brainstem. Over the centuries, a variety of other brain areas, including subregions of the prefrontal cortex (PFC), were identified by James Papez,[2] after whom this system was named as the *Papez circuit*, and Paul McLean,[3] who then called this functional pathway the "limbic system." The regions that form the limbic system include subcortical regions, comprising the olfactory bulb, hypothalamus (the endocrine part of the brain that responds to a variety of hormones), amygdala, mammillary bodies, nucleus accumbens, septum, and some thalamic nuclei, including the anterior dorsomedial nuclei, and cortical regions, comprising the hippocampal formation and regions of the neocortex, including the insular cortex, orbitofrontal cortex (OFC), cingulate gyrus, and parahippocampal gyrus (**Fig. 1**).

The limbic system is an evolutionary old brain system that plays an important role in learning and memory functions. It is also involved in the generation, integration, and

This work is supported by grant TP B3/SFB 779 from the German Science Foundation, and grants from the Bundesministerium für Bildung und Forschung (TUR 10/148) and the German-Israeli Foundation.

Department of Zoology and Developmental Neurobiology, Institute of Biology, Otto von Guericke University Magdeburg, Leipziger Street 44, Building 91, Magdeburg 39120, Germany

E-mail address: katharina.braun@ovgu.de

doi:10.1016/j.clp.2011.08.013
0095-5108/11/$ – see front matter © 2011 Elsevier Inc. All rights reserved.
perinatology.theclinics.com

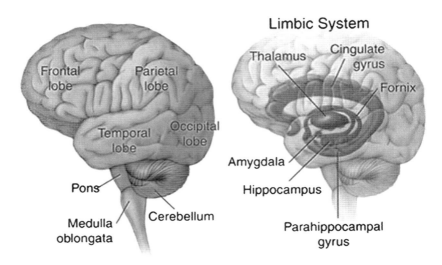

Fig. 1. Anatomic location of some limbic structures. (The medical illustration is provided courtesy of Alzheimer's Disease Research, a program of the American Health Assistance Foundation. © 2011.)

control of emotions, and connects them with the behavioral responses. For instance, the interpretation of facial expressions and the underlying emotional status of a person, or the evaluation of a dangerous situation and the decision to express an appropriate behavioral response (eg, fight-or-flight response), involves a variety of limbic brain regions, including the amygdala and prefrontal cortical regions. The limbic system is also tightly linked to the autonomic nervous system and, via the hypothalamus, interferes and regulates endocrine functions (eg, hormonal responses during stress). The amygdala, hippocampus, and medial PFC critically influence the responses of the hypothalamic-pituitary-adrenal (HPA) axis.[4,5] Furthermore, dysfunctions in these brain areas are implicated in the etiology of mental disorders, including depression and posttraumatic stress disorder, which are often characterized by HPA axis abnormalities,[6] and attention deficit-hyperactivity disorder (ADHD).[5,7]

The hippocampus (meaning *seahorse*) and dentate gyrus are essential for memory functions, especially memorizing facts and events. Damage to the hippocampus induces anterograde amnesia, causing the inability to form new memories, although old memories may still be intact. The hippocampus also plays an important role in spatial learning, and therefore is part of the brain's navigation system.

The amygdala (meaning *almond*) is connected to the PFC, hippocampus, septum, and dorsomedial thalamus. Because of its connectivity within the limbic system, it plays an important role in the mediation and control of emotions, including love and affection, fear, aggression, and reward, and therefore is essential for social behavior. For instance, damage to the amygdala reduces aggressive behavior and the experience of fear (ie, makes one less fearful), whereas electrical stimulation of the amygdala has the opposite effect.

The nucleus accumbens plays an important role in reward, pleasure, emotions (eg, laughter, crying), aggression, and fear. Of clinical relevance is its role in the pathologic form of reward (ie, addiction). The core and shell subregions of the nucleus accumbens receive inputs from a variety of limbic and prefrontal regions, including the amygdala and hippocampus to form a network that is involved in acquisition, encoding, and retrieval of aversive learning and memory processes.

The PFC can be roughly subdivided into (1) dorsolateral, (2) medial (which may include the functionally related anterior cingulate cortex), and (3) OFC (behind the eyes, or orbits).[8] Both the medial PFC and OFC are part of a frontostriatal circuit that has strong connections to the amygdala and other limbic regions. Thus, prefrontal regions are anatomically well suited to integrate cognitive and emotional functions.

The OFC is involved in sensory integration and higher cognitive functions, including decision making. The OFC also plays an essential role in a variety of emotional functions, such as judgment of the hedonic aspects of rewards or reinforcers, which is important for the planning of behavioral responses associated with reward and punishment. Dysfunction or damage to the OFC can result in poor empathy and impaired social interactions. The OFC also plays a major role in the regulation of aggression and impulsivity, and damage to the OFC leads to behavioral disinhibition, such as compulsive gambling, drug use, and violence.

The cingulate cortex can be cytoarchitectonically and functionally differentiated into an anterior part, which exerts executive functions, and a posterior part, which is evaluative. Furthermore, the cingulate cortex has two major subdivisions, a dorsal cognitive division and a rostral-ventral affective division.[9] A variety of studies indicate an anatomic and functional continuum rather than strictly segregated operations.[9,10] The ventral and dorsal areas of the cingulate cortex play a role in autonomic and a variety of rational cognitive functions, such as reward anticipation, decision-making, empathy, and emotional regulation.

DEVELOPMENT
The Concept of Experience-Expectant and Experience-Dependent Brain Development: Synaptic View

In the mammalian brain, including the human version, most functional neuronal pathways are optimized within the first 4 to 6 years of life, and this functional maturation is highly dependent on experience. The neonatal brain is programmed to be stimulated and excited by the environment; it is experience-expectant. This concept implies that perinatal experience (positive and adverse) exerts a much more pronounced impact on brain development than previously appreciated. Studies in animal models showed that the establishment and maintenance of functional neuronal networks in the developing brain are achieved through epigenetic changes, involving a complex, well-orchestrated interaction between genetic and environmental factors (**Fig. 2**). The genetic predisposition provides the individual framework within which social and cognitive behaviors and competences can develop. Throughout embryonic and postnatal brain development, sensory, motor, and emotional perceptions and the

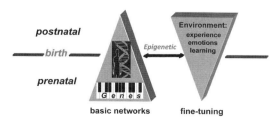

Fig. 2. Epigenetic mechanisms in brain development: interaction of genetic predisposition and environmental factors.

associated learning events activate or deactivate the genetic and molecular programs and thereby fine-tune and adapt functional neuronal networks to fit the individual's environment. Thus, the outcome of a given genetic predisposition can be positively influenced by adequate and stabilizing environmental factors, but it can also be influenced in an adverse direction in response to negative experience, inadequate stimulation, or deprivation. Visualizing the genome as a piano keyboard (see **Fig. 2**), the pianist represents the environment, and depending on which and how many keys are touched, the result will either be a highly complex symphony (reflecting a stimulating environment), a simple melody (reflecting a deprived environment), or chaos (reflecting inconsistent, random, and meaningless information from the environment). This example also illustrates that an excellent genetic predisposition does not automatically result in an optimally adapted and competent brain. Alternatively, genetic damage, such as Down syndrome or fragile X syndrome, which could be compared with broken keys on the keyboard, still has the potential to achieve remarkable capacities if the developing brain is provided with a stimulating environment.

On the neuronal level (**Fig. 3**), experience and learning about the cognitive and emotional aspects of the environmentally induce electrical, chemical (eg, dopamine, endogenous opiates, stress hormones), and, as a long-term consequence, structural (ie, synaptic rewiring) changes within prefronto-limbic neuronal networks. The unique characteristics of neonatal learning, which is also referred to with the ethological/ psychological term *imprinting*, is the fact that it occurs very fast and leaves lasting neuronal traces in the developing brain. Evidence is accumulating that cognitive and emotional concepts, behavioral skills, and strategies are shaped within the developing prefrontal and limbic system networks (see **Figs. 1** and **4**). The speed and stability of early learning events are most likely a product of the specific mechanisms

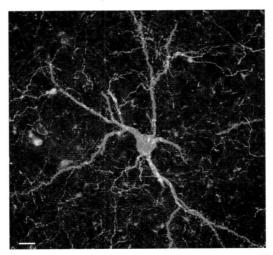

Fig. 3. Neuron (*red*) labeled with immunohistochemistry, using an antibody against dopamine- and cyclic AMP–regulated phosphoprotein with a molecular weight of 32 kDa (DARPP-32, a protein, which was discovered by Svenningsen and coworkers).[93] DARPP-32 is only expressed in neurons receiving dopaminergic input, which in this image are seen as green fluorescent fibers (*arrows*). The DARPP-32–expressing neuron displays numerous spine synapses (*ie, the small thorny protrusions*) and en-passant dopaminergic synapses (*seen as the double-labeled yellow structures*) on its dendrites. (*Courtesy of* Martin Metzger, University Sao Paolo, Brazil.)

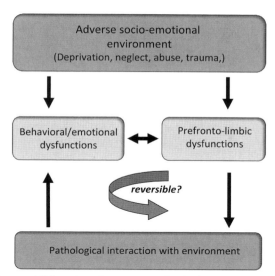

Fig. 4. Role of adverse childhood environment on brain development.

underlying juvenile learning. As opposed to adult learning, juvenile learning events may recruit additional neurodevelopmental mechanisms (see **Fig. 2**), which speed up the learning process. Because juvenile learning interferes with the ongoing development of neuronal functions, it dramatically affects synaptic reorganization resulting in long-term structural changes.[5,11] The main outcome of juvenile learning is most likely not primarily to collect and memorize facts and details, but rather to establish cognitive concepts, a "grammar" of emotionality and behavioral strategies, which critically determine behavior throughout life.

On the synaptic level, experience-expectant and experience-dependent brain maturation involve the proliferation and elimination of synaptic connections (see **Fig. 3**). Synaptic reorganization during brain development and during learning and memory formation follows the "use it or lose it" and "use it and improve it" principles and is guided by Hebb's[12] postulate that "neurons that fire together wire together." These mechanisms indicate that the establishment and maintenance of synaptic connections require a fine-tuned synchrony of neuronal activation. During the first years of life, the synapses compete against each other for survival, and only the synapses that are frequently activated survive, whereas less-active or silent synapses are weakened and eventually eliminated from the network. The pruning of synapses is an important mechanism in the developing brain that might be compared with the creation of a statue by removing material from the raw stone. However, although pruning involves the degeneration of chronically inactive synaptic connections, the author discovered that the elimination of abundant synapses is an activity-dependent process that is critically regulated by experience.[5,13] This experience-driven Darwinian synaptic reorganization[14] indicates that the capacity of the brain is primarily determined not by the quantity of its synaptic connections but rather by their quality and specificity.

The Concept of Experience-Expectant and Experience-Dependent Brain Development: Systemic View

In primates, including humans, the major brain systems are more or less functional at birth, even though they require adaptations and improvements of precision during postnatal development (see previous section). Sensory and motor systems (ie, visual, auditory, somatosensory, speech areas), and particularly higher cognitive and emotional systems such as the limbic and the prefrontal cortical systems, gradually optimize their functional capacity through experience- and learning-induced reorganization of neuronal networks. Different brain systems, however, do not mature all in parallel and at the same speed. Although the sensory systems develop early and, in humans, reach their full capacity during the first decade of life, the hippocampus and PFC (ie, regions that play an important role in higher cognitive tasks and memory functions) develop late and at a much slower pace.[15] The PFC (ie, the cortical region behind the forehead and is exceptionally large in primates) develops until the age of 20 years or longer in humans.

The pioneering neuroanatomic investigations of Huttenlocher and Dabolkar[16,17] and Rakic and colleagues[18] in human and nonhuman primates have clearly shown that each cortical region develops during a specific period of synaptic reorganization (see previous section). For each functional brain system, neuroscientists and developmental psychologists defined sensitive or critical phases of postnatal development. In the early studies of Arnold Scheibel,[19,20] Mark Rosenzweig,[21] and William Greenough[22] and their colleagues, the influence of differing environmental conditions on the development of sensory and motor cortices was experimentally analyzed in animal models. These experiments showed that early sensory or motor deprivation results in delayed or retarded maturation of synaptic connectivity in the affected cortical regions. For example, neurons in the visual cortex of rats, which were reared in the dark or in an impoverished environment, displayed significantly fewer synapses and smaller dendritic trees (the processes with the thorny protrusions illustrated in see **Fig. 3**) than neurons of rats, which were reared in a more complex and stimulating environment. Similar effects were found in the somatosensory and motor cortex of monkeys, which were reared in environments of different complexity.[23] The electrical and neurochemical properties and transduction mechanisms of neurons and synapses in the brain of humans, monkeys, and rats are identical, and because the experience-dependent maturation of brain functions follow common, evolutionary old mechanisms, similar developmental mechanisms likely also apply to the human brain.

Regions of the limbic system, such as the hippocampus, amygdala, nucleus accumbens, PFC, and cingulate gyrus, play distinct roles in cognitive and emotional development.[24] In humans and higher mammals, the differential maturation rates of the amygdala, septal nuclei, cingulate gyrus, and orbital frontal lobes seem to correspond to different phases of socioemotional development.[24] Joseph[24] and other authors proposed that the differential maturational rates of prefrontal and limbic nuclei, starting with the development of the amygdala and followed by the cingulate cortex and the septal nuclei, may be functionally linked to the observation that humans and other higher mammals as juveniles socialize indiscriminately, and only later form more selective emotional bonds. The maturational sequence of prefronto-limbic circuits may also be connected to the ability to express and experience emotions such as anger, joy, and fear of strangers, which emerges around the age of 6 months to 1 year.[24]

The human amygdala, which is involved in fear and anxiety, progresses and finalizes axonal myelination (ie, insulating neuronal axons with myelin to speed up the transmission of electrical signals along the axon) by the end of the first postnatal year. Researchers proposed that the indiscriminate socializing of the infant may be from the immaturity of the amygdala at this age, and that as functional maturation of the amygdala and its synaptic connections with other limbic and with prefrontal regions progresses, the infant starts to express a fear of strangers.[24] Between 1 and 3 years of age, a more selective strategy of socioemotional behavior emerges, and researchers suggested that this may also be linked to the maturation of the septum, which inhibits the indiscriminate social drive of the amygdala.[24] The human septal complex does not reach adult levels until 3 years of age, and its maturation continues into puberty.

The regions of the PFC exhibit considerable growth during early childhood, and their functional maturation lasts well into adolescence and adulthood. Postnatal development of the PFC includes the increase of metabolic and electrical activity,[25] which corresponds with synaptic reorganization[16,17] and progressing myelination.[26,27]

The human cingulate gyrus reaches an advanced stage of maturity during the first year, but continues to develop during the next several years. The extensive development of the connectivity of cingulate cortex from infancy to late childhood were proposed to correlate with behavioral development.[9] For instance, the reciprocal relationship between the cingulate's cognitive and emotional subdivisions, which continue to develop during early infancy, may underlie the observation in babies that signs of distress (including crying) can be blocked temporarily through orienting attention to an interesting object.[28,29] Moreover, evidence shows that abnormal development of the cingulate cortex and OFC is involved in the origin of major depressive mood disorders.

Between 4 to 18 years of age, sex-specific maturational changes were noted during postnatal development of the human amygdala and hippocampus volume. Although the left amygdala volume increases only in men, hippocampal volume increases only in women. This developmental pattern is most likely related to the distribution of sex hormone receptors in these limbic regions, with the amygdala predominantly expressing androgen receptors and the hippocampus predominantly expressing estrogen receptors.[30] Increasing evidence also shows that abnormal development of the amygdala and hippocampus may be involved in the origin of a variety of mental disorders. For instance, amygdala volumes are significantly larger in both hemispheres of patients with borderline personality disorder experiencing major depression compared with those without depressive symptoms.[31] In patients with bipolar disorder, a trend toward smaller volumes of the left amygdala was detected compared with control subjects; however, no significant differences were found in right amygdala volume or in right or left hippocampus.[32] Furthermore, brains of depressed suicide victims showed increased activity of output neurons in the right lateral amygdala,[33] and an elevated relative density of the glutamic acid decarboxylase-immunoreactive neuropil (indicating an increase in inhibition) was observed in the hippocampal formation.[34]

Impact of Perinatal Emotional Experience on Prefronto-Limbic Development

The concept of experience-expectant and experience-dependent brain development predicts that functional brain circuits, including the limbic system, require adequate and sufficient environmental stimulation, and that these circuits cannot achieve their full functional capacity under impoverished or otherwise adverse environmental conditions.[5,7,35] Although clinical and experimental animal studies showed the importance of early experience and learning in mental development, most studies have focused on the behavioral and endocrine level, and much less is known about the consequences of early experience and learning on structural and physiologic brain development. It is tempting to speculate that emotional templates, which are coded in the wiring of prefronto-limbic networks, are continuously modified during childhood, and again during adolescence, and determine emotional perception and regulation throughout life. Because of their slow developmental rate, prefrontal and limbic regions, which are essential for the maturation of emotional and cognitive competences, are exposed to an exceptionally long sensitive time window during which experience-dependent functional maturation can be modified. The neuroanatomic and functional connection between cognitive and emotional functions within prefronto-limbic pathways empha- sizes the importance of emotional experience during early childhood, which essen- tially shapes their function in adulthood. Of particular importance is the formation of a secure attachment and emotional bond between the child and the caregiver, which is formative for the child in developing an emotional language.

The cingulate gyrus, because of its connections with the OFC and the amygdala, plays an essential role in the establishment of the mother-infant attachment during the latter half of the first postnatal year, including the expression of maternal behavior and maternal separation anxiety in the infant.[36] In this context, the cingulate cortex plays a specific role in caregiver-infant attachment. The anterior cingulate cortex is part of the PANIC/GRIEF pathway, which has been described by Panksepp,[37] which is activated in the infant brain during separation stress. MacLean[38] and Lorberbaum and colleagues[36] proposed the thalamo-cingulate theory of parental behavior. Testing this hypothesis has shown that mothers display increased activity in the anterior cingulate and right medial PFC and other limbic regions while listening to their babies cry.[39,40] This baby-evoked activation is largely reduced in depressed mothers[41] and mothers who delivered through cesarean section.[42]

The author's studies in an animal model indicate that the infant-evoked activation of the maternal anterior cingulate cortex is mirrored by an activation of the infant's ante- rior cingulate cortex while listening to maternal vocalizations. When a newborn degu pup is separated from its family, the activity in the anterior cingulate cortex is down- regulated, but when the pup hears the mother's voice, the activity in these brain regions returns to almost normal levels.[43–45] The juvenile affection-evoked activation of the anterior cingulate cortex and other prefrontal and limbic structures seems to be maintained until adulthood. Functional MRI studies showed that adult students showed activation in the anterior cingulate cortex when shown pictures of romantic partners.[46] It is tempting to speculate that the parent-infant bond, representing the first love in one's life, teaches and entrains the developing brain regarding adult emotional experiences, including falling in love.

This emotional entrainment hypothesis implies that dysfunctional juvenile attach- ment may predispose an individual to develop lasting, and perhaps even irreversible impairment of, emotionality and social behavior later in life. Adverse (or the complete lack of) emotional experience can equally imprint in the brain and may result in retarded, dysfunctional synaptic wiring patterns, and these synaptic manifestations of traumatic memories may represent the neurologic substrate for the development of pathologic behaviors and mental disorders in humans. For instance, research has recently shown that the cingulate cortex is hypofunctional in aggressive children and teenagers[47] during emotional stimulation using the International Affective Picture System.

Experiments in a variety of animal models showed that stressful or traumatic events experienced during perinatal development, such as stress in utero or repeated or chronic separation from the parents, severely affect the structural and neurochemical development of the brain, particularly the maturation of the limbic system. This finding was first shown in the semi-precocious lagomorph *Octodon degus* (degu or trumpet- tailed rat), which displays closer similarities to human and nonhuman primates than the common laboratory rodents.[48] Degus live in social communities and a biparental family structure, they express the stress hormone cortisol, and their sensory systems are equally mature as those of human babies. Similar to human babies,[49] the neonate degu pups learn to recognize and respond to their mothers' vocalizations within the first days of life. Although common laboratory rodents do not seem to exhibit a filial attachment of the kind shown by young primates or humans, *Octodon degus* pups develop a strong attachment to both parents. Similar to humans, vocal communication between family members seems to be an essential component for the establishment and maintenance of their emotional attachment. The brain functional evidence for this attachment was detected using functional imaging techniques in 1-week old degus. During acute separation from the parents, the pups displayed significantly decreased metabolic activity in most limbic cortical and subcortical regions, and in some sensory cortical areas.[50]

The pioneering work of Meaney and colleagues[51–54] in laboratory rats emphasized the importance of maternal care in the development of neuronal and endocrine functions and behavior. They showed that adult offspring of high-licking and high-grooming mothers (ie, tactile somatosensory stimulation from caring mothers), compared with those from low-licking and low-grooming mothers (ie, neglecting mothers), had reduced adrenocorticotropic hormone and corticosterone (stress hormone) levels and reduced dendritic length and spine density in the hippocampus.[51,52] Researchers also found that offspring of "good" mothers displayed increased expression of N-methyl-D-aspartate receptor subunit and brain-derived neurotrophic factor mRNA, increased cholinergic innervation of the hippocampus, and enhanced spatial learning and memory.[53] Another study also showed that maternal behavior can stimulate synaptogenesis and simultaneously prevent neuronal cell death (apoptosis) in the hippocampus.[54] Using a mammalian imprinting model, Moriceau and colleagues[55] assessed the neural circuitry that enables infant rats to attach quickly to a caregiver using olfactory coding. Their work indicates that "the neonatal brain is not an immature version of the adult brain but is uniquely designed to optimize attachment to the caregiver."

Although most studies in humans and animal models have focused on the importance of maternal care and the mother-infant attachment, research is now beginning to assess the role of paternal care on brain development. The author's experiments in biparental *Octodon degus* showed striking differences in prefronto-limbic pathways between degus that were raised with both parents and those that were raised by a single mother. Father-deprived degus developed more shaft synapses (which can be excitatory or inhibitory) in the anterior cingulate cortex, fewer dendritic spines in the OFC (possibly indicating reduced excitatory activity in these brain regions), and longer dendrites in the basolateral amygdala (possibly reflecting elevated synaptic activity) compared with animals that were raised by both parents.[56,57] In addition to the excitatory synaptic changes, the expression of inhibitory neurons and of neurons that are part of the brain's stress system and express the stress hormone corticotropin-releasing hormone, and monoaminergic innervation of prefronto-limbic reward pathways, are significantly altered in father-deprived animals.[58,59] Some of these structural differences seem to be the result of delayed development because they normalize until adulthood, but others are stable and still evident in adulthood. In addition to the synaptic changes in the prefronto-limbic circuits, the father-deprived offspring developed fewer spine synapses in the somatosensory cortex,[60] which is the area where touch, temperature, and pain are perceived. This deprivation-induced reduction in synaptic connectivity seems likely to result from reduced body contact because of the lack of paternal care, emphasizing the importance of body contact in cortical development.

The critical impact on brain development of neonatal parental care and deprivation, respectively, implies that neglect and other adverse emotional experience, such as prenatal or postnatal stress, also may interfere with the development of prefrontal and limbic functions and perhaps leave permanent functional "scars" in these neuronal circuits. This view is supported by the findings in Romanian orphans, which showed that children undergo remarkable behavioral improvements when removed from orphanage settings and placed in family environments. However, long after adoption, these children still display deficits in emotional and social development.[61] Still, little is known about the processes through which early experiences of neglect lead to these developmental problems. Functional imaging studies showed that these children have prefrontal hypofunction.[62] They also seem to have enlarged right amygdala volumes, whereas the left amygdala volume was related to the time spent in institutions, with those experiencing longer periods of deprivation having a smaller left amygdala volume.[63]

Prefrontal and anterior cingulate hypofunction has also been diagnosed in patients with ADHD and schizophrenia, and in children, teenagers, and adults displaying pathologic or criminal aggression.[25,47,64–66] However, whether these brain differences are the result of experience-induced synaptic reorganization is unclear. To experimentally test the impact of prenatal or postnatal stress on neuronal and synaptic development, the author conducted several series of experiments in rats and degus. In 21- and 45-day-old degus, which were repeatedly exposed to daily parental separation during the first 3 weeks of life, they found significantly elevated densities of dendritic spine synapses (the thorny protrusions on the dendrites of the neuron shown in **Fig. 2**, which represent excitatory synapses) in the anterior cingulate cortex[67–69] and significantly elevated spine densities on hippocampal CA1 pyramidal neurons, whereas they saw significantly reduced spine densities on granule cell dendrites in the dentate gyrus and on apical dendrites of large pyramidal-shaped neurons in the medial nucleus of the amygdala.[69] In addition, the separation-stressed animals developed a dysbalance of inhibitory interneurons in prefrontal and limbic brain regions,[70,71] and also altered monoaminergic (serotonin, dopamine, noradrenaline) fiber innervation in these regions.[72–74] Imbalances of monoaminergc systems have also been found in monkeys reared in social isolation.[75]

These findings were replicated in laboratory rats, which can serve as a preterm baby model because of their immaturity at birth. To study a possible link between the synaptic changes and critical developmental time windows,[76] young rats were exposed to maternal separation at different ages. These experiments showed that the magnitude and direction of stress-induced synaptic changes depends on not only the brain region and cell type but also brain maturity at the time of stress exposure. Rats that experienced maternal separation stress between postnatal days 3 and 5 showed fewer dendritic spines in the anterior cingulate cortex, whereas pups that experienced the same degree of maternal separation during days 14 through 16 developed more spine synapses, which is comparable to the findings in degus.[76] Similar alterations were described in the amygdala of neonatally deprived rats, in which reduced numbers of perforated synapses and synaptic contact zones were found.

Stress exposure at an even earlier time window, such as stress in utero during the last week of gestation (ie, the pregnant dams were exposed to stress), showed highly sex-specific changes in neuronal morphology and synaptic density in the anterior cingulate and OFC[77] and in the hippocampus.[78] Neurons in the hippocampus of prenatally stressed male rats showed longer dendrites and more spine synapses, whereas their sisters showed the opposite effect.[78] In rats and humans, some of these (prenatal or postnatal) stress-induced neuronal changes can be reversed or prevented by daily handling (ie, applying tactile somatosensory stimulation).[78–80] Another example for the protective role of sensory-emotional stimulation was observed in degus, in which the author was able to show that stimulation with the voice of their mothers during separation can buffer and protect the pups' brains from stress-induced changes in dopaminergic and serotonergic receptors.[81,82]

In addition to the timing of stress exposure, brain region, neuron type, and gender, the intensity of the stressor also matters.[83] Testing mild, high, or no-stress from gestational days 12 through 16 in rats showed significantly different and often opposite effects in behavioral and brain development. Mild prenatal stress decreased brain weight in both males and females, whereas extreme stress increased female brain weight. Mild prenatal stress slowed the development of sensorimotor abilities and decreased locomotion, whereas high prenatal stress also slowed development of sensorimotor learning but increased locomotion. Furthermore, the "flavor" of stress also seems to matter for the neonatal developing brain. Exposure to a daily injection of isotonic saline (which may be compared with the routine blood sampling in the neonatology/neonatal intensive care unit facilities) induces a dramatic loss of dendritic spine synapses in the anterior cingulate cortex, which is the opposite synaptic effect of what has been found after maternal separation stress (C. Helmeke, PhD, unpublished data, 2000).

These experience-induced changes in behavior, neuronal morphology, and synaptic density are not restricted to rodents. Monkeys that were raised in isolation displayed severe behavioral abnormalities,[84–86] and their brains showed reduced dendritic complexities and synaptic densities in the motor cortex.[87] Even though much more extensive research is required, similar structural changes seem likely to occur in the human brain in response to perinatal emotional experience.

CONCLUSIONS AND CLINICAL IMPLICATIONS

Extensive research on mother-infant interactions has shown convincing evidence that the early conversations between parent and child laid the basis for cognitive, emotional, and communicative and linguistic development. During the prelinguistic period, babies are capable of expressing a behavioral repertoire in relation to the capacity of their internal brain activity, which stimulates the reciprocal relation with corresponding brain activity of the caregivers.[88,89] Even though the behavioral expressions for communicating are still very immature at birth, they are powerful enough to enter an affective communication system, in which the infant's goal-directed strivings are aided and supplemented by the capacities of the caretaker. The caretaker interprets these messages and adapts actions to facilitate the infant's intensions. In preterm babies, this behavioral repertoire is much less developed because of the immaturity of their brains, and therefore they are not yet fully equipped to enter the dialog with their caregivers.

This immaturity of the communicative systems in particular involves the late-developing prefronto-limbic pathways, which mediate cognitive and emotional competences and are thus essential for communicating. The immaturity of these systems must be considered with respect to the concept of experience-expectant and experience-dependent development of the brain and behavior, because neonatal cognitive and emotional experience have been shown to be essential for the functional maturation of PFC and limbic brain circuits. At birth the brain mainly acts via a brain-stem regulatory system interconnected with limbic regions, such as the amygdala and hippocampus, which are all reciprocally connected with the PFC where synaptic reorganization is starting to undergo epigenetic sculpting. Particularly for the preterm and neonate infant, emotional stimulation represents a major critical input into the infant's brain, which triggers the first neonatal learning event, the formation of an emotional attachment to the caregivers.

The human brain is programmed to express and receive emotions, which before speech development enter the infant's brain via different sensory systems. The sensory systems of babies are already functional, but they have to undergo experience-dependent optimization during specific sensitive time windows. The olfactory system, which has the closest synaptic connection to the limbic system, processes olfactory cues, such as the smell of maternal/paternal skin, which are used to identify the caregiver. The auditory system interprets the prosodic aspects of the caretakers' child-directed speech ("motherese") into emotional signals, but it is also activated and can be overstimulated by loud or continuous noise (just as the visual system may be overstimulated by bright light), which may lead to habituation and reduced sensitivity toward emotional acoustic signals. The somatosensory system conducts tactile stimulation experienced during body contacts with the caregiver, but it is also activated by painful stimulations, such as blood drawing and intubation. The immaturity of the sensory systems in the preterm baby limits the complexity of the incoming signals from the environment, and thereby impairs the communicative dialog between the child and the caretakers. The sensory cues from the environment enter the prefronto-limbic pathways in the infant's brain, where they are translated into emotional information and thereby train emotional behavioral responses in the infant. Again, the immaturity of the preterm baby's motor control limits the complexity of its behavioral responses to communicate with the caregivers. This early emotional training seems to be critical for adult emotionality, because the neuronal substrate underlying emotional behavior is shaped and optimized early in life, and the studies in Romanian orphans clearly indicate that this emotional repertoire and "grammar" seems to remain very stable throughout life. Because the limbic system is also essential for cognitive functions, learning, and memory, it seems likely that inappropriate or deprivation of emotional stimulation during early childhood may also result in cognitive impairments, such as delayed speech learning and other skills. More detailed research is required to better understand the functional interconnections between the immature sensory and prefronto-limbic pathways in preterm babies to develop optimal ways to communicate with the infant and thereby provide emotional and cognitive stimulation that is adequate to the capacity of the child's brain.

A host of research in animal models has studied the impact of stress on the brain; however, most studies have focused on the effects of chronic stress on the adult brain.[6] The author's own studies on the impact of separation- and pain-associated stress in the immature, prenatal, and neonatal preterm rodent brain showed that the neuronal and synaptic outcome in the PFC and limbic regions strongly depends on the maturity of the brain systems involved in stress coping at the time of stress exposure, the gender of the brain, and the type and duration of stress.[5,65,77,78,90] Convincing evidence shows that at least part of these neuronal and synaptic changes are mediated by glucocorticoid stress hormones.[5,90] This finding raises the important question of whether and in which way steroids with glucocorticoid properties, such as dexamethasone, which is frequently used in preterm babies with bronchopulmonary dysplasia to improve pulmonary function,[91] may interfere with neuronal and synaptic development. Animal research has shown that chronic exposure to corticosteroids results in decreased brain weight, impaired cell division, delayed cortical dendritic branching, and disrupted glial cell formation. More detailed research is required to asses whether these drug treatment–induced changes in neural cell division and differentiation are permanent and irreversible, and how these currently unavoidable treatments may be replaced by better therapies with fewer side effects.

Clinical and animal research has shown the critical importance of developmentally sensitive time windows. Although for the sensory systems (visual, auditory, somatosensory) the opening and closing of developmental time windows are well defined, the PFC and limbic regions develop later and more slowly, leaving a long time window open for experience-driven optimization. This extended sensitive time window also provides an elevated vulnerability toward adverse environmental influences, which may result in irreversibly impaired neuronal development. Thus, preventative and therapeutic interventions should be undertaken as early as possible and within these critical developmental periods to take advantage of the elevated neuronal and synaptic plasticity of these time windows, not only to accelerate therapeutic effects but also to achieve long lasting repairs.

It is also becoming evident from studies on neuronal regeneration in humans and in animal models after brain injuries that experience-dependent mechanisms are essentially involved in neuronal and synaptic repair.[92] Preterm babies have a specifically high risk of brain damage, which, if not treated early and with appropriate therapies, may become irreversible. In addition to the initial efforts to limit the severity of the injury to minimize loss of function, timely efforts are required to reorganize the brain to restore and compensate for function that has already been lost or compromised in its development. Again, most research on regenerative neuronal mechanisms and therapies have focused on brain damage in the adult brain. The developing brain is a moving target for interventions and therapies because of its progressing maturation. So far not enough is known about the temporal dynamics of neuronal differentiation and synaptic development that occur in the preterm brain, which is a brain that is not yet fully equipped to handle the world outside of the mother's womb. Thus, because of the immaturity of the preterm infant's brain, whether a therapeutic intervention is appropriate or may cause even more severe damage is difficult to assess. However, the immature brain has a much higher plasticity for reorganizing synaptic connections, which have just started to form. Along these lines, research has shown that a common outcome of brain damage is that individuals spontaneously develop compensatory behavioral strategies that can drive experience-induced reorganization of synaptic connectivity in and among affected brain regions. Thus, a brain that is exposed to rehabilitative training may have already reorganized itself through compensatory behavioral changes. These self-taught behavioral changes can be adaptive and support the functional outcome of therapies, and, ideally in the immature brain, timely therapeutic interventions should assist and complement this self-organizing healing process. However, the self-regulated rehabilitation can also be maladaptive and interfere with or even prevent intervention-induced improvements in function, particularly if the latter are applied at a later developmental stage of the (then-less-plastic) brain. Although considerable knowledge exists about regenerative mechanisms after injuries of sensory and motor functions (eg, loss of vision, speech, hearing, movement of limbs) and the underlying neuronal reorganization, much less is known about the neuronal mechanisms underlying emotional rehabilitation. Furthermore, because of the limited capacity of preterm babies to express themselves, the degree and direction of spontaneously occurring compensatory behaviors is much more difficult to assess.

SUMMARY

The knowledge that neonatal emotional experience and associated learning processes are critical in the maturation of prefronto-limbic circuits emphasizes the great responsibility and importance of preterm and neonatal care. The further improvement of care and intervention strategies requires the detailed understanding of epigenetic mechanisms of neuronal and synaptic reorganization underlying the emergence of emotional and cognitive behavioral traits. The best way to get there is to stimulate (and fund) interdisciplinary research efforts in which pediatricians and developmental biologists and psychologists merge their knowledge, concepts, and methodology. The hope is that in the future the translational relevance of research efforts can be improved through a greater interaction between basic and clinical scientists, which also should improve the awareness of basic neuroscientists of the problems faced by those in the clinic who are administering preterm and neonatal care.

REFERENCES

1. Broca P. Anatomie comparée des circonvolutions cérébrales: le grand lobe limbique. Rev Anthropol 1878;1:385–498.
2. Papez JW. A proposed mechanism of emotion. Arch Neurol Psychiatr 1937;38: 725–43.
3. Maclean PD. Some psychiatric implications of physiological studies on frontotemporal portion of limbic system (visceral brain). Electroencephalogr Clin Neurophysiol 1952;4(4):407–18.
4. Herman JP, Ostrander MM, Mueller NK, et al. Limbic system mechanisms of stress regulation: hypothalamo-pituitary-adrenocortical axis. Prog Neuropsychopharmacol Biol Psychiatry 2005;29:1201–13.
5. Bock J, Braun K. The impact of perinatal stress on the functional maturation of prefronto-cortical synaptic circuits: implications for the pathophysiology of ADHD? Prog Brain Res 2011;189:155–69.
6. McEwen BS, Magarinos AM. Stress effects on morphology and function of the hippocampus. Ann N Y Acad Sci 1997;821:271–84.
7. Bush G. Cingulate, frontal, and parietal cortical dysfunction in attention-deficit/ hyperactivity disorder. Biol Psychiatry 2011;69(12):1160–7.
8. Happaney K, Zelazo PD, Stuss DT. Development of orbitofrontal function: current themes and future directions. Brain Cogn 2004;55:1–10.
9. Bush G, Luu P, Posner MI. Cognitive and emotional influences in anterior cingulate cortex. Trends Cogn Sci 2000;4(6):215–22.
10. Mohanty A, Engels S, Herrington JD, et al. Differential engagement of anterior cingulate cortex subdivisions for cognitive and emotional function. Psychophysiology 2007;44:343–51.
11. Comery TA, Shah R, Greenough WT. Differential rearing alters spine density on medium-sized spiny neurons in the rat corpus striatum: evidence for association of morphological plasticity with early response gene expression. Neurobiol Learn Mem 1995;63:217–9.
12. Hebb DO. The organization of behavior: a neuropsychological theory. New York: Wiley; 1949.
13. Segal M. Dendritic spines and long-term plasticity. Nat Rev Neurosci 2005;6(4): 277–84.
14. Changeux JP, Danchin A. Selective stabilisation of developing synapses as a mechanism for the specification of neuronal networks. Nature 1976;264: 705–12.
15. Chugani HT. Biological basis of emotions: brain systems and brain development. Pediatrics 1998;102(5 Suppl E):1225–9.
16. Huttenlocher PR. Synaptic density in human frontal cortex—developmental changes and effects of aging. Brain Res 1979;163:195–205.
17. Huttenlocher PR, Dabholkar AS. Regional differences in synaptogenesis in human cerebral cortex. J Comp Neurol 1997;387:167–78.
18. Rakic P, Bourgeois JP, Goldman-Rakic PS. Synaptic development of the cerebral cortex: implications for learning, memory, and mental illness. Prog Brain Res 1994;102:227–43.

19. Scheibel ME, Lindsay RD, Tomiyasu U, et al. Progressive dendritic changes in aging human cortex. Exp Neurol 1975;47:392–403.
20. Scheibel ME, Lindsay RD, Tomiyasu U, et al. Progressive dendritic changes in the aging human limbic system. Exp Neurol 1976;53:420–30.
21. Rosenzweig MR, Bennett EL. Psychobiology of plasticity: effects of training and experience on brain and behavior. Behav Brain Res 1996;78:57–65.
22. Turner AM, Greenough WT. Differential rearing effects on rat visual cortex synapses. I. Synaptic and neuronal density and synapses per neuron. Brain Res 1985;329:195–203.
23. Bryan GK, Riesen AH. Deprived somatosensory-motor experience in stumptailed monkey neocortex: dendritic spine density and dendritic branching of layer IIIB pyramidal cells. J Comp Neurol 1998;286:208–17.
24. Joseph R. Environmental influences on neural plasticity, the limbic system, emotional development and attachment: a review. Child Psychiatry Hum Dev 1999;29(3):189–208.
25. Rubia K, Overmeyer S, Taylor E, et al. Hypofrontality in attention deficit hyperactivity disorder during higher-order motor control: a study with functional MRI. Am J Psychiatry 1999;156:891–6.
26. Pfefferbaum A, Mathalon DH, Sullivan EV, et al. A quantitative magnetic resonance imaging study of changes in brain morphology from infancy to late adulthood. Arch Neurol 1994;51(9):874–87.
27. Yakovlev PJ, Lecours AR. The myelogenetic cycles of regional maturation of the brain. In: Minskowski A, editor. Regional development of the brain in early life. Oxford (United Kingdom): Blackwell; 1967. p. 3–10.
28. Harman C, Rothbart MK, Posner MI. Distress and attention interactions in early infancy. Motiv Emot 1997;21:27–43.
29. Posner MI, Rothbart MK. Attention, self regulation and consciousness. Philos Trans R Soc Lond B Biol Sci 1998;353:1915–27.
30. Giedd J, Vaituzis C, Hamburger SD, et al. Quantitative MRI of the temporal lobe, amygdala, and hippocampus in normal human development: ages 4-18 years. J Comp Neurol 1996;366:223–30.
31. Zetzsche T, Frodl T, Preuss UW, et al. Amygdala volume and depressive symptoms in patients with borderline personality disorder. Biol Psychiatry 2006; 60(3):302–10.
32. Chen BK, Sassi R, Axelson D, et al. Cross-sectional study of abnormal amygdala development in adolescents and young adults with bipolar disorder biol. Psychiatry 2004;56:399–405.
33. Gos T, Krell D, Bielau H, et al. Demonstration of disturbed activity of the lateral amygdaloid nucleus projection neurons in depressed patients by the AgNOR staining method. J Affect Disord 2010;126(3):402–10.
34. Gos T, Günther K, Bielau H, et al. Suicide and depression in the quantitative analysis of glutamic acid decarboxylase-immunoreactive neuropil. J Affect Disord 2009;113(1–2):45–55.
35. Black JE, Greenough WT. Developmental approaches to the memory process. In: Martinez JL Jr, Kesner RP, editors. Neurobiology of learning and memory. San Diego (CA): Academic Press, Inc; 1998. p. 55–88.
36. Lorberbaum JP, Newman JD, Horwitz AR, et al. A potential role for thalamocingulate circuitry in human maternal behavior. Biol Psychiatry 2002;51(6):431–45.
37. Panksepp J, Watt D. Why does depression hurt? Ancestral primary-process separation-distress (PANIC/GRIEF) and diminished brain reward (SEEKING) processes in the genesis of depressive affect. Psychiatry 2011;74(1):5–13.

38. MacLean PD. Triune brain in evolution: role in paleocerebral functions. New York: Plenum Press; 1990.

39. Numan M, Sheehan TP. Neuroanatomical circuitry for mammalian maternal behavior. Ann N Y Acad Sci 1997;807:101–25.

40. Leckman JF, Herman AE. Maternal behavior and developmental psychopathology. Biol Psychiatry 2002;51(1):27–43.

41. Laurent HK, Ablow JC. A cry in the dark: depressed mothers show reduced neural activation to their own infant's cry. Soc Cogn Affect Neurosci, 2011. [Epub ahead of print].

42. Swain JE, Tasgin E, Mayes LC, et al. Maternal brain response to own baby-cry is affected by cesarean section delivery. J Child Psychol Psychiatry 2008;49: 1042–52.

43. Poeggel G, Braun K. Early auditory filial learning in degus (Octodon degus): behavioral and autoradiographic studies. Brain Res 1996;743:162–70.

44. Braun S, Scheich H. Influence of experience on the representation of the "mothering call" in frontoparietal and auditory cortex of pups of the rodent Octodon degus: FDG mapping. J Comp Physiol A 1997;181(6):697–709.

45. Braun K, Poeggel G. Recognition of mother's voice evokes metabolic activation in the medial prefrontal cortex and thalamus of Octodon degus pups. Neuroscience 2001;103:861–4.

46. Bartels A, Zeki S. The neural basis of romantic love. Neuroreport 2000;11(17): 3829–34.

47. Stadler C, Sterzer P, Schmeck K, et al. Reduced anterior cingulate activation in aggressive children and adolescents during affective stimulation: association with temperament traits. J Psychiatr Res 2007;41(5):410–7.

48. Colonnello V, Iacobuccia P, Fuchs T, et al. Octodon degus. A useful animal model for social-affective neuroscience research: basic description of separation distress, social attachments and play. Neurosci Biobehav Rev 2011;35:1854–63.

49. DeCasper AJ, Fifer WP. Of human bonding: newborns prefer their mother's voices. Science 1980;208:1174–6.

50. Braun K, Bock J. Early traumatic experience alters metabolic brain activity in thalamic, hypothalamic and prefrontal cortical brain areas of Octodon degus. Dev Psychobiol 2003;43(3):248.

51. Champagne DL, Bagot RC, van Hasselt F, et al. Maternal care and hippocampal plasticity: evidence for experience-dependent structural plasticity, altered synaptic functioning, and differential responsiveness to glucocorticoids and stress. J Neurosci 2008;28(23):6037–45.

52. Bagot RC, van Hasselt FN, Champagne DL, et al. Maternal care determines rapid effects of stress mediators on synaptic plasticity in adult rat hippocampal dentate gyrus. Neurobiol Learn Mem 2009;92(3):292–300.

53. Liu D, Diorio J, Day JC, et al. Maternal care, hippocampal synaptogenesis and cognitive development in rats. Nat Neurosci 2000;3:799–806.

54. Weaver IC, Grant RJ, Meaney MJ. Maternal behavior regulates long-term hippocampal expression of BAX and apoptosis in the offspring. J Neurochem 2002;82: 998–1002.

55. Moriceau S, Roth TL, Sullivan RM. Rodent model of infant attachment learning and stress. Dev Psychobiol 2010;52(7):651–60.

56. Ovtscharoff W Jr, Helmeke C, Braun K. Lack of paternal care affects synaptic development in the anterior cingulate cortex. Brain Res 2006;1116:58–63.

57. Helmeke C, Seidel K, Poeggel G, et al. Paternal deprivation during infancy results in dendrite- and time-specific changes of dendritic development and spine

formation in the orbitofrontal cortex of the biparental rodent Octodon degus. Neuroscience 2009;63:790–8.

58. Seidel K, Holetschka R, Poeggel G, et al. Paternal deprivation alters the development of corticotropin releasing factor (CRF)-expressing neurons in the orbitofrontal cortex, amygdala and hippocampus of the biparental rodent Octodon degus. J Neuroendocrinology, 2011. [Epub ahead of print].

59. Braun K, Seidel K, Weigel S, et al. Paternal deprivation alters region- and age-specific interneuron expression patterns in the biparental rodent Octodon degus. Cereb Cortex 2011;21:1532–46.

60. Pinkernelle J, Abraham A, Helmeke C, et al. Paternal deprivation induces dendritic and synaptic changes and hemispheric asymmetry of pyramidal neurons in the somatosensory cortex. Dev Neurobiol 2009;69:663–73.

61. O'Connor TG, Rutter M. Attachment disorder behavior following early severe deprivation: extension and longitudinal follow-up. English and Romanian Adoptees Study Team. J Am Acad Child Adolesc Psychiatry 2000;39:703–12.

62. Chugani HT, Behen ME, Muzik O, et al. Local brain functional activity following early deprivation: a study of postinstitutionalized Romanian orphans. Neuroimage 2001;14:1290–301.

63. Mehta MA, Golembo NI, Nosarti C, et al. Amygdala, hippocampal and corpus callosum size following severe early institutional deprivation: the English and Romanian Adoptees study pilot. J Child Psychol Psychiatry 2009;50:943–51.

64. Raine A, Buchsbaum M, LaCasse L. Brain abnormalities in murderers indicated by positron emission tomography. Biol Psychiatry 1997;42:495–508.

65. Brower MC, Price BH. Neuropsychiatry of frontal lobe dysfunction in violent and criminal behaviour: a critical review. J Neurol Neurosurg Psychiatry 2001;71:720–6.

66. Manoach DS. Prefrontal cortex dysfunction during working memory performance in schizophrenia: reconciling discrepant findings. Schizophr Res 2003;60: 285–98.

67. Helmeke C, Ovtscharoff W Jr, Poeggel G, et al. Juvenile emotional experience alters synaptic composition in the anterior cingulate cortex. Cereb Cortex 2001; 11:717–27.

68. Helmeke C, Poeggel G, Braun K. Differential emotional experience induces elevated spine densities on basal dendrites of pyramidal neurons in the anterior cingulate cortex. Neuroscience 2001;104:927–31.

69. Poeggel G, Helmeke C, Abraham A, et al. Juvenile emotional experience alters synaptic composition in the rodent cortex, hippocampus, and lateral amygdala. Proc Natl Acad Sci U S A 2003;100:16137–42.

70. Seidel K, Helmeke C, Kindler J, et al. Repeated neonatal separation stress alters the composition of neurochemically characterized interneuron subpopulations in the rodent dentate gyrus and basolateral amygdala. Dev Neurobiol 2008;68: 1137–52.

71. Helmeke C, Ovtscharoff W Jr, Poeggel G, et al. Imbalance of immunohistochemically characterized interneuron populations in the adolescent and adult rodent medial prefrontal cortex after repeated exposure to neonatal separation stress. Neuroscience 2008;152:18–28.

72. Braun K, Lange E, Metzger M, et al. Maternal separation followed by early social deprivation affects the development of monoaminergic fiber systems in the medial prefrontal cortex of Octodon degus. Neuroscience 2000;95:309–18.

73. Poeggel G, Nowicki L, Braun K. Early social deprivation alters monoaminergic afferents in the orbital prefrontal cortex of Octodon degus. Neuroscience 2003; 116:617–20.

74. Gos T, Becker K, Bock J, et al. Early neonatal and postweaning social emotional deprivation interferes with the maturation of serotonergic and tyrosine hydroxylase- immunoreactive afferent fiber systems in the rodent nucleus accumbens, hippocampus and amygdala. Neuroscience 2006;140:811–21.

75. Martin LJ, Spicer DM, Lewis MH, et al. Social deprivation of infant rhesus monkeys alters the chemoarchitecture of the brain: I. Subcortical regions. J Neurosci 1991;11:3344–58.

76. Bock J, Gruss M, Becker S, et al. Experience-induced changes of dendritic spine densities in the prefrontal and sensory cortex: correlation with developmental time windows. Cereb Cortex 2005;15:802–8.

77. Murmu MS, Salomon S, Biala Y, et al. Changes of spine density and dendritic complexity in the prefrontal cortex in offspring of mothers exposed to stress during pregnancy. Eur J Neurosci 2006;24:1477–87.

78. Bock J, Murmu MS, Biala Y, et al. Prenatal stress and neonatal handling induce sex-specific changes in dendritic complexity and dendritic spine density in hippocampal subregions of prepubertal rats. Neuroscience 2011;193:34–43.

79. Schanberg SM, Field TM. Sensory deprivation stress and supplemental stimulation in the rat pup and preterm human neonate. Child Dev 1987;58:1431–47.

80. van Oers HJ, de Kloet ER, Whelan T, et al. Maternal deprivation effect on the infant's neural stress markers is reversed by tactile stimulation and feeding but not by suppressing corticosterone. J Neurosci 1998;18:10171–9.

81. Ziabreva I, Poeggel G, Schnabel R, et al. Separation-induced receptor changes in the hippocampus and amygdala of Octodon degus: Influence of maternal vocalizations. J Neurosci 2003;23:5329–36.

82. Ziabreva I, Schnabel R, Poeggel G, et al. Mother's voice "buffers" separation-induced receptor changes in the prefrontal cortex of Octodon degus. Neuroscience 2003;119:433–41.

83. Mychasiuk R, Ilnytskyy S, Kovalchuk O, et al. Intensity matters: brain, behaviour and the epigenome of prenatally stressed rats. Neuroscience 2011;180:105–10.

84. Harlow HF, Harlow MK. Social deprivation in monkeys. Sci Am 1962;207:137–46.

85. Suomi SJ. Early determinants of behaviour: evidence from primate studies. Br Med Bull 1997;53:170–84.

86. Suomi SJ. Early stress and adult emotional reactivity in rhesus monkeys. Ciba Found Symp 1991;156:171–88.

87. Struble RG, Riesen AH. Changes in cortical dendritic branching subsequent to partial social isolation in stumptailed monkeys. Dev Psychobiol 1978;11:479–86.

88. Trevarthen C. Communication and cooperation in early infancy: a description of primary intersubjectivity. In: Bullowa M, editor. Before speech: the beginning of interpersonal communication. New York: Cambridge University Press; 1979. p. 321–47.

89. Tronick E. Emotions and emotional communication in infants. Am Psychol 1989; 44(2):112–9.

90. Bock J, Braun K. Blockade of N-methyl-D-aspartate receptor activation suppresses learning-induced synaptic elimination. Proc Natl Acad Sci U S A 1999; 96(5):2485–90.

91. Ng PC. The effectiveness and side effects of dexamethasone in preterm infants with bronchopulmonary dysplasia. Arch Dis Child 1993;68:330–6.

92. Kleim JA, Jones TA. Principles of experience-dependent neural plasticity: implications for rehabilitation after brain damage. J Speech Lang Hear Res 2008; 51:225–39.

93. Svenningsson P, Nishi A, Fisone G, et al. DARPP-32: an integrator of neurotransmission. Annu Rev Pharmacol Toxicol 2004;44:269–96.

Epigenetic Effects of Early Developmental Experiences

Kathryn M.A. Gudsnuk, Frances A. Champagne, PhD*

KEYWORDS

- Epigenetic pathway • Postnatal maternal care
- DNA methylation

Experiences occurring in early development can exert long-term effects that lead to either heightened or attenuated risk of physical and psychiatric disease. Of particular importance for these outcomes is the quality of the relationship between a parent and an infant. Parental stress, reduced sensitivity of parents to infant cues, and childhood neglect/abuse may lead to a cascade of biological changes that compromise the functioning of infants, leading to effects that persist into adolescence and adulthood. Moreover, genetic and environmental factors may heighten the vulnerability of infants to these effects. For the high-risk neonate, both underlying vulnerability and adverse early-life experiences are characteristic and may ultimately lead to divergent developmental pathways that compromise future health and well-being. The deprivation or reduction in parental contact that is often experienced by these infants during the neonatal period may be a significant factor in determining the severity of these outcome measures. Thus, understanding the mechanisms through which parental care can alter infant development may provide insight into the potential interventions and practices that are critical in promoting healthy children, adolescents, and adults.

During fetal and infant development, the brain is rapidly changing, leading to proliferation and refinement of neural pathways. The sensitive period created by this time of neuronal plasticity creates a window of opportunity during which experiences can exert long-term effects. Although the study of human brain development and the effects of experiences on these processes has been limited by the availability of appropriate methodological tools, decades of work using animal models has provided some valuable insights. Laboratory studies of rodents suggest that adverse experiences occurring during fetal and/or infant development lead to changes in brain architecture and function. These effects are particularly evident when the quality of the parent-infant interaction is affected, either through parental stress or through

Department of Psychology, Columbia University, Room 406 Schermerhorn Hall, 1190 Amsterdam Avenue, New York, NY 10027, USA
* Corresponding author.
E-mail address: fac2105@columbia.edu

Clin Perinatol 38 (2011) 703–717
doi:10.1016/j.clp.2011.08.005
0095-5108/11/$ – see front matter © 2011 Published by Elsevier Inc.

manipulation of the quality and/or quantity of parental care toward infants. More recent approaches to the study of the mechanism of parental effects have determined that in addition to physiologic and neurobiological outcomes, the quality of the parent-infant interactions may induce a molecular change in offspring, which alters the patterns of gene expression present in specific brain regions. These epigenetic effects indicate that the quality of the early-life environment can change the activity of genes, thus illustrating the dynamic interplay between genes and environmental experiences in shaping development.

This article highlights research that has investigated the epigenetic mechanisms which may contribute to the lasting psychobiological impact of early-life adversity. In particular, the authors focus on studies that demonstrate the impact of maternal stress, variation in parental care, parental deprivation, and infant abuse on the epigenetic pathways. Although primarily drawn from work with laboratory rodents, there is increasing evidence for similar effects in human infants, and this new and emerging evidence is explored. The implications of this research are significant and may provide insight into those features of the early environment that may exert profound effects on the developing brain. The authors speculate as to the way in which this research can inform neonatal practices and provide strategies for improving the care of high-risk infants.

EPIGENETIC PATHWAYS: A PRIMER

The pathways through which DNA exerts a biological effect that leads to variation in physiology, metabolism, and behavior are being increasingly explored using modern techniques from molecular biology. An emerging theme from this work is the dynamic ways in which DNA is regulated by a variety of factors, leading to variation in the expression or activity of genes. Within the cell nucleus, DNA is stored in a highly compact and densely coiled configuration, a strategy that is necessary for storing the billions of nucleotide base pairs in the mammalian genome. For genes to have a biological impact, they must be expressed. Gene expression involves the transcription of DNA into messenger RNA, which is then translated into protein (**Fig. 1**A). The transcription of DNA is a very elegant process, and the timing and level of gene expression are critical for the normal process of development. The mechanisms that are capable of altering gene expression without altering gene sequence are called epigenetic, meaning over or above genetic.[1] Epigenetic mechanisms are typically molecular changes to the DNA itself or to the proteins around which the DNA is tightly coiled. In the context of environmentally induced epigenetic changes, most research has focused on posttranslational histone modifications and DNA methylation.

Within the cell nucleus, DNA is wrapped around histone proteins, and this wrapping allows for the compact storage of the genetic material.[2] However, the expression/activation of genes requires that the DNA become liberated from this dense structure and accessible to transcription factors and other enzymes, such as RNA polymerase, that initiate the transcription process (see **Fig. 1**B). One way to achieve this outcome is to modify the histone proteins so that they are less attracted to the DNA. Histone proteins possess extensions or tails that, when wrapped around the DNA, serve to reduce accessibility of the gene sequence. The addition of chemicals to or removal of chemicals from these histone tails can dynamically change the interaction between histones and DNA. For example, histone acetylation is a process whereby an acetyl chemical is added to the histone protein tail. When this occurs, there is typically increased gene expression because of a looser interaction between the histones and the DNA (see **Fig. 1**C). In contrast, removal of acetyl chemicals from histone tails (deacetylation) results in reduced gene expression. There are many chemicals that can be added

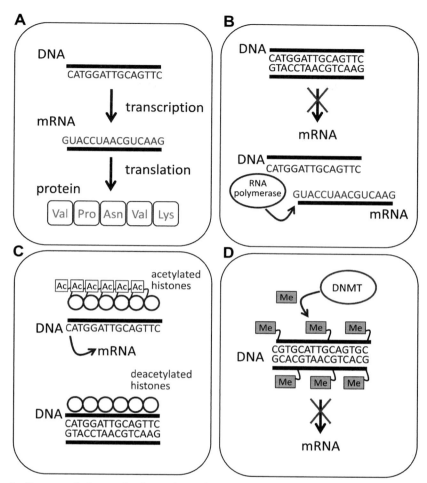

Fig. 1. Gene regulation and epigenetic mechanisms. (*A*) The activity of genes is determined by the level of transcription of DNA to messenger RNA (mRNA). The process of translation involves the use of mRNA to generate a protein consisting of a succession of amino acids. (*B*) When DNA is tightly compact (*top*), there is a suppression of gene expression (ie, no mRNA is produced). When DNA is less compact (*bottom*), enzymes such as RNA polymerase can bind to the DNA and initiate the process of transcription. (*C*) The addition of an acetyl chemical (Ac) to histone proteins can loosen the interactions between histones and DNA and increase the level of gene transcription (*top*). In contrast, deacetylated histones can be found to cluster closely to the DNA and suppress gene expression (*bottom*). (*D*) DNA methylation is a process in which methyl chemicals (Me) are added to cytosines in the DNA sequence by the enzyme DNMT. Methylated DNA is highly compact, and DNA methylation leads to reduced gene expression or gene silencing.

to or removed from the histone tails (a process generally called posttranslational modification) such that histones can undergo phosphorylation, methylation, and ubiquitination and multiple other chemical modifications.[3] Collectively, these modifications are called the histone code.[4] The interpretation of this code is complex, and these histone modifications represent a dynamic and complex strategy for reducing or enhancing gene expression.

A second epigenetic process of critical importance for development is DNA methylation. The addition of a methyl chemical to cytosines within the DNA strand represents a more stable and enduring epigenetic modification. When cytosines become methylated, there is generally less accessibility to the DNA, and consequently, DNA methylation is thought to be a process that leads to gene silencing (see **Fig. 1**D).[5] Moreover, methylated DNA can attract methyl-binding proteins that cluster around the DNA and attract enzymes that can shift the histone tails into a deacetylated state (further reducing access to the DNA).[6] A feature of DNA methylation that makes this epigenetic mechanism particularly intriguing is the potential heritability of DNA methylation patterns. When cells divide, they reliably copy their DNA material such that each cell within an organism contains the same DNA. A cell's DNA methylation patterns are also copied during the process of cell division. During cellular differentiation, the reliable transmission of DNA methylation patterns from mother to daughter cells is critical.[7,8] The diversity of cell types within one's body is generated through this epigenetic process, leading, for example, to the formation of differentiated neurons, blood cells, and muscle cells, which are identical in genetic information but differ significantly in epigenetic profiles. Thus, the epigenetic character of a cell, by determining the pattern of gene expression, determines the phenotype or character of the cell.

During the fetal and neonatal periods of life, there are rapid changes occurring within the developing organism that require the proliferation and differentiation of cells. The profound importance of epigenetic modifications during this time is highlighted by the effects of disruptions to the enzymes that are necessary for posttranslational histone modifications and DNA methylation. Studies using mice with a targeted deletion of a histone acetyltransferase gene indicate that disruption to this enzyme can be lethal and also associated with deficits in neural tube closing.[9] In the case of DNA methylation, the enzymes that are critical for this process are known as DNA methyltransferases (DNMTs). DNMT1 is a subtype of DNMT classified as a maintenance methyltransferase, which alludes to the role of this enzyme in maintaining the methylation patterns of cells after DNA replication/cell division. In contrast, DNMT3a and DNMT3b are called de novo methyltransferases and are thought to be primarily involved in adding new methyl chemicals to the unmethylated DNA.[10] Deletion of DNMT1 is associated with genome-wide hypomethylation, whereas overexpression of this gene leads to DNA hypermethylation, and both these genetic manipulations induce embryonic lethality.[11,12] Growth and survival are similarly impaired in DNMT3a/DNMT3b mutants.[13] Thus, activation of epigenetic pathways is essential for successful development.

EPIGENETIC PERSPECTIVES OF THE BIOLOGICAL IMPACT OF THE EARLY ENVIRONMENT

Our understanding of the biological significance of epigenetic variation is expanding rapidly. The dynamic, yet potentially stable changes in epigenetic regulation of gene expression that have been observed have raised intriguing questions: Could these mechanisms explain the effect of early-life experiences? Are epigenetic pathways a link between our experiences and the biobehavioral consequences of those experiences? Although initially it was assumed that plasticity of epigenetic modification was limited to the very early embryonic stages of development, this assumption has been challenged by the increasing evidence for environmentally induced epigenetic variation across the life span.[14] Variation in early-life exposure to toxins, nutritional levels, hormones, stress, and social interactions, which have been demonstrated to exert long-term effects on the brain, is also being demonstrated to be associated with histone modifications and changes in DNA methylation across the genome and within target genes. Although we are still unclear regarding the mechanisms that permit this level of plasticity within epigenetic pathways, the implications of these epigenetic effects are far reaching. The following sections highlight the investigations of the epigenetic effects associated with prenatal maternal stress/distress, postnatal maternal care, and neglect or abuse in early infancy. These studies serve to illustrate the profound impact that parent-offspring interactions can have on molecular, physiologic, neurobiological, and behavioral outcomes.

PRENATAL MATERNAL STRESS EFFECTS ON EPIGENETIC VARIATION AND INFANT DEVELOPMENT

Stress during pregnancy has been implicated as a significant risk factor for various fetal outcomes and developmental disorders. In humans, the experience of a severe stressor during gestation, such as exposure to a natural disaster or terrorist attack, has been associated with preterm birth, reduced birth weight, and a smaller head circumference.[15,16] Similarly, maternal anxiety and depression have been associated with obstetric complications and preterm birth.[17,18] The long-term consequences of prenatal stress in humans have also been documented and suggest that increased risk of schizophrenia and depression may be linked to this form of early-life adversity.[19] Although it is presumed that fetal exposure to elevated levels of stress hormones in maternal circulation is etiologically relevant to these outcomes, our understanding of the mechanism of prenatal stress effects is drawn primarily from laboratory studies using rodents. In these studies, pregnant rats or mice are exposed to a variety of stressors during gestation, and offspring development, neurobiology, and behavior are assessed. In general, these studies confirmed the short- and long-term effects of maternal stress that have been observed in humans and also indicated that maternal glucocorticoids are a mediating factor for these outcomes.[20,21] In addition, changes in gene expression are associated with exposure to prenatal stress, and these changes in gene activity can persist into adulthood. As such, there is potential for the involvement of epigenetic pathways in these prenatal effects.

In mice, exposure to chronic variable stress during pregnancy has been used to model prenatal adversity and has been found to exert sex-specific long-term neurobiological effects.[22] In particular, this early-life exposure induces changes in the stress response pathways, primarily involving the hypothalamic-pituitary-adrenal (HPA) response to stress. Within the HPA pathways, an external stressor leads to neuronal activation within the hypothalamus, which triggers the release of corticotropin-releasing factor (CRF) and vasopressin. CRF and vasopressin then stimulate the release of adrenocorticotropic hormone (ACTH) from the pituitary gland. The ACTH then stimulates the release of glucocorticoids (cortisol in humans and corticosterone in rodents) from the cortex of the adrenal gland. The glucocorticoids proceed to induce physiologic changes in several tissues, leading to the psychobiological changes we associate with the experience of stress: increased heart rate, blood pressure, and abnormalities in sleep-wake rhythms.[23] Although these short-term effects are often adaptive, increasing alertness and vigilance in response to threat, prolonged exposure to glucocorticoids may induce detrimental effects such as immunosuppression, weight gain, and depressed mood. To prevent the long-term exposure to glucocorticoids, there is a negative feedback loop that acts on the HPA axis involving glucocorticoid receptors (GRs) in the hippocampus. Glucocorticoid stimulation of these receptors triggers an inhibition of hypothalamic and pituitary release of CRF and ACTH, leading to reduced stimulation of glucocorticoid output from the adrenal gland.[24] Thus, there are both stress-enhancing and stress-inhibiting brain regions and receptor/hormone targets that can be considered when exploring the mechanism through which stress during pregnancy can lead to stress sensitivity in later life.

The epigenetic consequences of chronic variable stress in mice have been examined in several target genes, including CRF and GR. In male pups born to a stressed dam, CRF gene expression is increased and GR gene expression is decreased in adulthood.[22] These changes in gene activity likely account for the increased corticosterone release to stress and increased depression-like behavior that is observed among stressed males. Quantification of DNA methylation within the promoter region of these genes (a region of DNA that is critical for gene regulation) indicates that prenatal stress is associated with decreased DNA methylation of the CRF gene promoter and increased methylation of the GR promoter region in hypothalamic tissue of adult male offspring. The direction of these epigenetic effects coincides well with the notion that increased DNA methylation leads to reduced gene expression. When considering the mechanism of prenatal effects, it is important to consider the functioning of the placenta, a tissue in which dysregulation of gene expression has been found associated with intrauterine growth retardation in humans.[25] In the context of the study of chronic variable stress effects in mice, placental gene expression is altered by gestational stress, with particular effects on DNMT1.[22] Thus, there may be widespread epigenetic variation within the placenta consequent to this early-life exposure.

Although the translation of this work to the study of human prenatal adversity is challenging because of the limited accessibility to tissues and reduced control over moderating and mediating variables (such as nutrition, smoking, and intensity/timing of stressors), there is increasing evidence for epigenetic variation associated with maternal mood. Depression during pregnancy is associated with increased maternal cortisol level and reduced gestational length and thus shares some common features with stress exposure during pregnancy.[26] Analysis of cord blood samples from infants born to mothers with elevated ratings of depression (using the Hamilton Depression Scale) during the third trimester of pregnancy indicates elevated levels of DNA methylation within the GR promoter region.[27] The degree of DNA methylation within the neonatal GR promoter was found to predict increased salivary cortisol levels in infants at 3 months of age. In a recent study, the persistence of these prenatal effects on GR methylation was highlighted.[28] Children and adolescents (aged 10–19 years) born to women who had experienced stress in the form of intimate partner violence during pregnancy were found to have elevated GR methylation levels in whole blood samples. Although the interpretation of the meaning of these epigenetic changes in blood has yet to be fully elucidated, these findings support the hypothesis of lasting epigenetic variation in response to prenatal adversity.

EPIGENETIC CONSEQUENCES OF POSTNATAL MATERNAL CARE

Variation in the quality and/or quantity of mother-infant interactions has been demonstrated across several species, including humans,[29] and is increasingly being explored as a route through which individual differences in physiology and behavior emerge. This variation can be induced by the quality of the environment, and maternal stress and depression are significant predictors of the quality of postnatal mother-infant interactions.[30,31] In particular, the level of tactile stimulation (gentle touching and stroking) that mothers provide to infants is predicted by maternal mood (eg, depressed mothers provide less tactile stimulation). The tactile context of human caregiving has been demonstrated to influence pain sensitivity, affect, and growth in neonates.[32] Increasing awareness of the advantages of touch for infant development has led to changes in neonatal practices, such as encouragement of kangaroo care, skin-to-skin contact, and infant massage. These practices may be most advantageous for high-risk preterm infants, and when mothers are involved in the contact, the reciprocal tactile stimulation between mother and infant may contribute to increased maternal responsiveness and infant attachment.[32,33]

The biological impact of mother-infant interactions has been explored in laboratory rodents, and findings suggest that there are natural variations in maternal care in rodents that predict variation in offspring neurobiological and behavioral measures.[34] Rodents provide tactile stimulation to offspring through licking/grooming of pups (LG, a stimulation that can be mimicked by stroking with a paintbrush), and comparison of Long-Evans rat pups that have received low levels of LG with pups that have received high levels of LG has yielded valuable insights into the molecular and epigenetic factors that are shaped by maternal care. Maternal LG has been found to influence HPA reactivity, cognition, and reproductive behavior of offspring.[35] Analysis of the GR levels in the hippocampus of low LG male offspring compared with high LG offspring indicates that increased LG level is associated with increased hippocampal GR level in adulthood.[36] Consistent with this finding, offspring of high LG dams seem to have enhanced negative feedback of the HPA response to stress and have reduced corticosterone and ACTH levels after a stressor. Within the promoter region of the hippocampal GR gene, offspring of low LG dams have increased DNA methylation compared with offspring of high LG dams.[37] This differential methylation is not evident prenatally and emerges during the first week postpartum, a time during which LG behavior is at its peak among high LG dams. Histone acetylation and binding of transcription factors to the GR promoter region were also found to be increased among the offspring of high LG dams.[37] Within the hippocampus of low LG offspring, there are also reduced levels of glutamic acid decarboxylase (GAD1), the rate-limiting enzyme in γ-aminobutyric acid synthesis. Analysis of the GAD1 promoter region suggests that maternal LG induces a decrease in DNA methylation of this gene associated with increases in histone acetylation at this region.[38] Although most of these analyses have been conducted in male offspring, among the female offspring, the experience of low levels of LG during the postnatal period has been found to be associated with decreased transcription of estrogen receptor alpha (ERα) in the medial preoptic area of the hypothalamus (MPOA) and elevated DNA methylation within the promoter region of this gene.[39,40] Maternal effects on ERα DNA methylation and transcription may account for the effects of maternal care on reproductive/maternal behavior of female offspring.[41] Cross-fostering studies confirm that these epigenetic effects on gene expression are associated with the quality of the care received in infancy.

The impact of tactile stimulation during infancy on epigenetic pathways has also been explored using supplementary stimulation of rat pups using a paintbrush to provide licking-like stroking. Among artificially reared pups (ie, pups reared in the absence of the mother), the provision of a minimal level of tactile stimulation is necessary for survival and increasing the frequency of this stimulation during the neonatal period can significantly ameliorate the deficits induced by isolation from the mother.[42,43] Tactile stimulation in rodents is thought to influence sexual dimorphism in neuronal circuits, and there is evidence for sex differences in DNA methylation of the ERα promoter region in the MPOA.[44] Males have been demonstrated to have higher levels of ERα DNA methylation in this brain region compared with females. If females are provided with additional tactile stimulation during postnatal days 5 to 7, there are increases in DNA methylation of ERα such that females become indistinguishable from males regarding the methylation of this gene. Previous studies have demonstrated that male pups are licked more frequently than female pups during the postnatal period,[45] and it may be that this stimulation triggers epigenetic pathways that enhance sex differences in the brain. Enhanced tactile stimulation of pups can also be induced by using a communal nesting paradigm in which multiple females provide care for the neonates.[46] Mouse pups reared in these conditions have been found to have increased histone acetylation at the brain-derived neurotrophic factor (BDNF) gene promoter and, like offspring that have been reared by high LG dams, manifest numerous neurobiological and behavioral effects of this enriched early experience.[47,48] Although maternal care certainly provides stimulation of multiple sensory systems, tactile stimulation provided by mothers to infants can have long-term epigenetic consequences, and these findings complement the growing literature on the hormonal, physiologic, and behavioral effects of human touch.[32]

EPIGENETIC EFFECTS OF ABUSE AND NEGLECT

In light of the impact of natural variations in maternal care on epigenetic pathways, extreme forms of postnatal experience, such as neglect or abuse, would likewise be predicted to induce changes in gene activity. Maternal separation studies on laboratory primates and rodents have been used as a strategy to model early maternal deprivation/neglect and have demonstrated the causal influence of this form of early-life adversity on multiple neuroendocrine and behavioral outcomes. Similar to the effects of prenatal stress and low levels of maternal care, studies using mice in which pups are repeatedly separated from the mother during infancy indicate increased corticosterone secretion in response to stress.[49] Consistent with the role of hypothalamic vasopressin (AVP) within the HPA axis, maternal separation–induced stress sensitivity is associated with increased hypothalamic expression of the AVP gene in adult mice. DNA methylation levels within key regulatory regions of the AVP gene were found to differ between control (normally reared) and maternally separated offspring, with decreased AVP DNA methylation among maternally separated male offspring.[49] This hypomethylation of the AVP gene was also associated with reduced levels of binding of MeCP2 (a methyl-binding protein). Separation-induced effects on epigenetic alterations within the serotonin transporter (5-HTT) gene have likewise been demonstrated. Among rhesus macaques and humans, there is genetic variation within the 5-HTT promoter that has been associated with variation in risk or resilience to stressors such as childhood maltreatment.[50,51] Rhesus macaques that are reared in conditions of maternal separation and possess the risk allele of the 5-HTT gene were found to have increased DNA methylation of 5-HTT gene in blood cells.[52] Thus, there are interactions between genetic variation and epigenetic effects in response to early-life adversity, and these interactions may be an important consideration when predicting the degree of impact of maternal neglect in infancy.

Childhood abuse is a significant predictor of long-term physical and psychiatric disorder and a major public health concern. Similar to maternal neglect, the experience of maternal abuse can be modeled in laboratory rodents to determine the causal impact of this experience on the developing brain. Among laboratory rats, reduction in nesting materials provided to lactating dams during the postnatal period significantly increases the incidence of aggressive encounters between pups and dams (such as stepping on pups, aggressive grooming, and transporting of pups by a limb) and decreases the frequency of nurturing behaviors such as LG.[53,54] When pups are exposed to caregivers (nonbiological mothers) that are provided with limited nesting materials and placed in an unfamiliar environment, there is increased exposure of pups to these aggressive behaviors. The epigenetic consequence of these experiences has been determined for the BDNF gene in the prefrontal cortex.[55] Post-natal maltreatment predicts reduced expression of BDNF in the prefrontal cortex in adulthood. Among nonabused offspring, there are very low levels of DNA methylation within the BDNF gene promoter, whereas abused offspring have elevated levels of this repressive epigenetic modification. BDNF plays a critical role in brain development and neuronal plasticity.[56] Thus, reductions in BDNF achieved through epigenetic silencing of this gene may account for the profound effect of childhood maltreatment and lead to heightened risk of psychopathology among abused children.

The relevance of these epigenetic effects for childhood abuse in humans has been high-lighted in a study that analyzed postmortem brain tissue.[57] Gene expression and DNA methylation analyses were conducted with brain tissue from suicide victims with or without a documented history of childhood abuse and a control non-suicide comparison group. GR expression in the hippocampus was found to be equivalent among controls and suicide victims without a history of abuse, whereas a history of abuse predicted reduced GR expression. DNA methylation analysis of this gene indicated that, consistent with the gene expression findings, DNA methylation within the GR promoter region was low and equivalent between controls and nonabused suicide victims, whereas childhood abuse was associated with increased DNA methylation and decreased transcription factor binding within the GR gene promoter. The consistency of these findings with the rodent work is clear and suggests that epigenetic mechanisms may play a general role across species in encoding information regarding the experiences of an individual (**Fig. 2**).

Although no direct relationship can be established between the literature on child abuse and neglect and early experiences of high-risk neonates, it is conceivable that the nature of the infant's early birth or congenital problems, painful and unpredict-able procedures, inconsistency with pain alleviating and soothing interventions, and separation from the regulating processes of the mother contribute to early changes in brain with potential epigenetic consequences. Moreover, children who have disabil-ities, similar to those of preterm infants with a documented risk for later developmental delay, are reported to be referred to child protective services more frequently than children who do not have disabilities.[58–60]

EPIGENETICS AND PLASTICITY: IMPLICATIONS FOR INTERVENTION

Although we have much to learn about the processes through which our experiences can shape gene activity, studies of epigenetic variation in response to the quality of the prenatal and postnatal environment illustrate the potential plasticity of these mecha-nisms. Moreover, the responsivity of these pathways to variation in parental stress or postnatal mother-infant interactions suggests that interventions focused on moder-ating these aspects of the environment could have a significant impact on our biology. Studies on rodents suggest that maternal stress during gestation can lead to signifi-cant reductions in maternal care toward offspring,[61] and the occurrence of this phenomenon in humans is suggested by the effects of maternal stress and depressed mood on the frequency and quality of mother-infant interactions. Thus, an intervention targeted at alleviating maternal stress or mood may have significant downstream consequences for infant development. Increasing parental sensitivity to infant cues and promoting increased caregiver contact with infants may also be an effective strategy for intervention.[62] Studies of severely neglected infants suggest that adoption into foster families can ameliorate deficits in functioning.[63,64] These findings are com-plemented by animal studies in which enrichment during juvenile development can ameliorate the deficits associated with prenatal or postnatal adversity.[65–67]

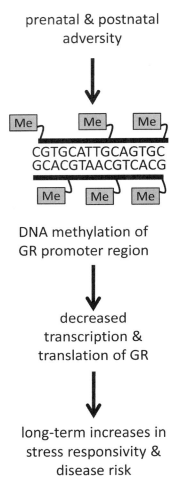

prenatal & postnatal
adversity

DNA methylation of
GR promoter region

decreased
transcription &
translation of GR

long-term increases in
stress responsivity &
disease risk

Fig. 2. Summary of the epigenetic effects of adversity on GRs. Studies on humans and rodents provide evidence for prenatal and postnatal adversity (maternal stress, low levels of postnatal infant care, and childhood abuse) on DNA methylation of the GR gene promoter. Increased adversity is associated with increased GR methylation and decreased expression of this gene. Consequently, exposed individuals have a heightened response to stress, leading to increased risk of the disease (physical and psychiatric).

Plasticity is a phenomenon typically associated with the early stages of development, and like most biological processes, changeability of epigenetic modifications may decline over developmental time. However, this phenomenon does not suggest that epigenetic effects are unchangeable in later life. In the case of the epigenetic consequences of variation in maternal LG levels, pharmacologic targeting of the epigenome has been used to reverse the effects of postnatal maternal care on gene expression, physiology, and behavior. Adult males that had been reared by low LG dams were found to have decreased GR promoter DNA methylation, increased hippocampal GR expression, and reduced corticosterone response to stress if treated with a drug that induced histone acetylation.[37] In contrast, if adult offspring of high LG dams are treated with a drug that increases the amount of methyl donors (methyl chemicals that can potentially methylate the DNA), these offspring are found to have increased GR promoter DNA methylation, decreased GR expression, and heightened stress reactivity.[68] This epigenetic plasticity is likely not limited to pharmacologic interventions, and the change in epigenetic profiles over time and in response to early- and later-life experiences will certainly be an interesting phenomenon to explore in both human and animal studies.

FUTURE DIRECTIONS IN THE STUDY OF EPIGENETICS AND INFANT DEVELOPMENT

For the high-risk neonate, issues regarding parental stress and deprivation of parental contact are very meaningful. Although the biological effects of nutritional or sensory deprivation may be well established, the quality of the early social/tactile environment can likewise have a lasting effect. Continued efforts to minimize the separation between mothers and infants during the postnatal period and to enhance the quality of mother-infant interactions when they occur are likely to ameliorate some of the effects of the early-life adversity to which these infants are exposed. An emerging theme within studies of epigenetic effects of the environment concerns the implications of these effects for subsequent generations of offspring. The heritability of DNA methylation patterns is certainly a critical feature of this epigenetic mark in the context of cellular differentiation. Recent studies suggest that environmentally induced epigenetic variation may also be inherited by offspring and grand-offspring generations.[69] For example, maternal separation in mice has been found to induce DNA methylation changes in the male germline, and similar epigenetic variation is observed in the brains of the offspring of these maternally separated males.[70] Epigenetic modifications may also be transmitted over generations through the stable transmission of maternal behavior from one generation to the next.[71] Taken together, these studies suggest that the consequences of perinatal experiences may not be limited to the individual experiencing adversity but may also be observed in the nonexposed offspring of these individuals. A multigenerational perspective in future studies of high-risk neonates may prove to be informative of the mechanisms through which infants and their families are influenced by these experiences.

Although the translation of laboratory studies of epigenetic effects has certainly made progress, there is much to be gained from continued study of epigenetic variation in humans. Similar to studies on rhesus macaques, there is evidence for genetic-epigenetic-experience interactions in humans, which predict biobehavioral outcomes,[72,73] and examining these interactions in response to the specific experiences of high-risk infants would be particularly informative. Longitudinal studies involving noninvasive measures of epigenetic variation over time would likewise enhance our understanding of the pathways through which the quality of the environment shapes our brain and behavior. As our basic understanding of epigenetic mechanisms expands and techniques for studying these mechanisms become more readily available and feasible to implement, there is increasing promise that an epigenetic perspective can be applied to the study of infant development. This perspective combined with the measures of neurobiological and behavioral function would allow for a depth of understanding of the development of high-risk neonates that spans from molecular to neurobiological and psychological functioning; a depth that may give rise to more refined and targeted interventions to enhance infant and parent well-being.

REFERENCES

1. Jablonka E, Lamb MJ. The changing concept of epigenetics. Ann N Y Acad Sci 2002;981:82–96.

2. Turner B. Chromatin and gene regulation. Oxford (United Kingdom): Blackwell Science Ltd; 2001.
3. Peterson CL, Laniel MA. Histones and histone modifications. Curr Biol 2004; 14(14):R546–51.
4. Jenuwein T, Allis CD. Translating the histone code. Science 2001;293(5532): 1074–80.
5. Razin A. CpG methylation, chromatin structure and gene silencing—a three-way connection. EMBO J 1998;17(17):4905–8.
6. Fan G, Hutnick L. Methyl-CpG binding proteins in the nervous system. Cell Res 2005;15(4):255–61.
7. Fukuda S, Taga T. Cell fate determination regulated by a transcriptional signal network in the developing mouse brain. Anat Sci Int 2005;80(1):12–8.
8. Jones PA, Taylor SM. Cellular differentiation, cytidine analogs and DNA methylation. Cell 1980;20(1):85–93.
9. Bu P, Evrard YA, Lozano G, et al. Loss of Gcn5 acetyltransferase activity leads to neural tube closure defects and exencephaly in mouse embryos. Mol Cell Biol 2007;27(9):3405–16.
10. Turek-Plewa J, Jagodzinski PP. The role of mammalian DNA methyltransferases in the regulation of gene expression. Cell Mol Biol Lett 2005;10(4):631–47.
11. Biniszkiewicz D, Gribnau J, Ramsahoye B, et al. Dnmt1 overexpression causes genomic hypermethylation, loss of imprinting, and embryonic lethality. Mol Cell Biol 2002;22(7):2124–35.
12. Jackson-Grusby L, Beard C, Possemato R, et al. Loss of genomic methylation causes p53-dependent apoptosis and epigenetic deregulation. Nat Genet 2001;27(1):31–9.
13. Okano M, Bell DW, Haber DA, et al. DNA methyltransferases Dnmt3a and Dnmt3b are essential for de novo methylation and mammalian development. Cell 1999;99(3):247–57.
14. Champagne FA. Epigenetic influence of social experiences across the lifespan. Dev Psychobiol 2010;52(4):299–311.
15. Hobel CJ, Goldstein A, Barrett ES. Psychosocial stress and pregnancy outcome. Clin Obstet Gynecol 2008;51(2):333–48.
16. Dancause KN, Laplante DP, Oremus C, et al. Disaster-related prenatal maternal stress influences birth outcomes: Project Ice Storm. Early Hum Dev 2011. [Epub ahead of print].
17. Alder J, Fink N, Bitzer J, et al. Depression and anxiety during pregnancy: a risk factor for obstetric, fetal and neonatal outcome? A critical review of the literature. J Matern Fetal Neonatal Med 2007;20(3):189–209.
18. Field T, Diego M, Hernandez-Reif M, et al. Comorbid depression and anxiety effects on pregnancy and neonatal outcome. Infant Behav Dev 2010;33(1):23–9.
19. Schlotz W, Phillips DI. Fetal origins of mental health: evidence and mechanisms. Brain Behav Immun 2009;23(7):905–16.
20. Barbazanges A, Piazza PV, Le Moal M, et al. Maternal glucocorticoid secretion mediates long-term effects of prenatal stress. J Neurosci 1996;16(12): 3943–9.
21. Weinstock M. The long-term behavioural consequences of prenatal stress. Neurosci Biobehav Rev 2008;32(6):1073–86.
22. Mueller BR, Bale TL. Sex-specific programming of offspring emotionality after stress early in pregnancy. J Neurosci 2008;28(36):9055–65.
23. Stratakis CA, Chrousos GP. Neuroendocrinology and pathophysiology of the stress system. Ann N Y Acad Sci 1995;771:1–18.

24. Sapolsky RM, Meaney MJ, McEwen BS. The development of the glucocorticoid receptor system in the rat limbic brain. III. Negative-feedback regulation. Brain Res 1985;350(1–2):169–73.

25. McMinn J, Wei M, Schupf N, et al. Unbalanced placental expression of imprinted genes in human intrauterine growth restriction. Placenta 2006;27(6–7): 540–9.

26. O'Keane V, Lightman S, Marsh M, et al. Increased pituitary-adrenal activation and shortened gestation in a sample of depressed pregnant women: a pilot study. J Affect Disord 2011;130(1–2):300–5.

27. Oberlander TF, Weinberg J, Papsdorf M, et al. Prenatal exposure to maternal depression, neonatal methylation of human glucocorticoid receptor gene (NR3C1) and infant cortisol stress responses. Epigenetics 2008;3(2):97–106.

28. Radtke KM, Ruf M, Gunter HM, et al. Transgenerational impact of intimate partner violence on methylation in the promoter of the glucocorticoid receptor. Transl Psychiatry 2011;1:e21.

29. Hane AA, Fox NA. Ordinary variations in maternal caregiving influence human infants' stress reactivity. Psychol Sci 2006;17(6):550–6.

30. Field T. Postpartum depression effects on early interactions, parenting, and safety practices: a review. Infant Behav Dev 2010;33(1):1–6.

31. Field T. Early interactions between infants and their postpartum depressed mothers. Infant Behav Dev 2002;25(1):25–9.

32. Field T. Touch for socioemotional and physical well-being: a review. Dev Rev 2010;30:367–83.

33. Bystrova K, Ivanova V, Edhborg M, et al. Early contact versus separation: effects on mother-infant interaction one year later. Birth 2009;36(2):97–109.

34. Meaney MJ. Maternal care, gene expression, and the transmission of individual differences in stress reactivity across generations. Annu Rev Neurosci 2001;24: 1161–92.

35. Cameron NM, Champagne FA, Parent C, et al. The programming of individual differences in defensive responses and reproductive strategies in the rat through variations in maternal care. Neurosci Biobehav Rev 2005;29(4–5):843–65.

36. Liu D, Diorio J, Tannenbaum B, et al. Maternal care, hippocampal glucocorticoid receptors, and hypothalamic-pituitary-adrenal responses to stress. Science 1997;277(5332):1659–62.

37. Weaver IC, Cervoni N, Champagne FA, et al. Epigenetic programming by maternal behavior. Nat Neurosci 2004;7(8):847–54.

38. Zhang TY, Hellstrom IC, Bagot RC, et al. Maternal care and DNA methylation of a glutamic acid decarboxylase 1 promoter in rat hippocampus. J Neurosci 2010;30(39):13130–7.

39. Champagne FA, Weaver IC, Diorio J, et al. Maternal care associated with methylation of the estrogen receptor-alpha1b promoter and estrogen receptor-alpha expression in the medial preoptic area of female offspring. Endocrinology 2006;147(6):2909–15.

40. Champagne FA, Weaver IC, Diorio J, et al. Natural variations in maternal care are associated with estrogen receptor alpha expression and estrogen sensitivity in the medial preoptic area. Endocrinology 2003;144(11):4720–4.

41. Champagne FA. Maternal imprints and the origins of variation. Horm Behav 2011; 60(1):4–11.

42. Gonzalez A, Lovic V, Ward GR, et al. Intergenerational effects of complete maternal deprivation and replacement stimulation on maternal behavior and emotionality in female rats. Dev Psychobiol 2001;38(1):11–32.

43. Lovic V, Fleming AS. Artificially-reared female rats show reduced prepulse inhibition and deficits in the attentional set shifting task—reversal of effects with maternal-like licking stimulation. Behav Brain Res 2004;148(1–2):209–19.

44. Kurian JR, Olesen KM, Auger AP. Sex differences in epigenetic regulation of the estrogen receptor-alpha promoter within the developing preoptic area. Endocrinology 2010;151(5):2297–305.

45. Moore CL, Morelli GA. Mother rats interact differently with male and female offspring. J Comp Physiol Psychol 1979;93(4):677–84.

46. Curley JP, Davidson S, Bateson P, et al. Social enrichment during postnatal development induces transgenerational effects on emotional and reproductive behavior in mice. Front Behav Neurosci 2009;3:25.

47. Branchi I, Karpova NN, D'Andrea I, et al. Epigenetic modifications induced by early enrichment are associated with changes in timing of induction of BDNF expression. Neurosci Lett 2011;495(3):168–72.

48. Branchi I. The mouse communal nest: investigating the epigenetic influences of the early social environment on brain and behavior development. Neurosci Biobehav Rev 2009;33(4):551–9.

49. Murgatroyd C, Patchev AV, Wu Y, et al. Dynamic DNA methylation programs persistent adverse effects of early-life stress. Nat Neurosci 2009;12(12):1559–66.

50. Caspi A, Sugden K, Moffitt TE, et al. Influence of life stress on depression: moderation by a polymorphism in the 5-HTT gene. Science 2003;301(5631):386–9.

51. Aguilera M, Arias B, Wichers M, et al. Early adversity and 5-HTT/BDNF genes: new evidence of gene? Environment interactions on depressive symptoms in a general population. Psychol Med 2009;39(9):1425–32.

52. Kinnally EL, Capitanio JP, Leibel R, et al. Epigenetic regulation of serotonin transporter expression and behavior in infant rhesus macaques. Genes Brain Behav 2010;9:575–82.

53. Ivy AS, Brunson KL, Sandman C, et al. Dysfunctional nurturing behavior in rat dams with limited access to nesting material: a clinically relevant model for early-life stress. Neuroscience 2008;154:1132–42.

54. Raineki C, Moriceau S, Sullivan RM. Developing a neurobehavioral animal model of infant attachment to an abusive caregiver. Biol Psychiatry 2010;67(12):1137–45.

55. Roth TL, Lubin FD, Funk AJ, et al. Lasting epigenetic influence of early-life adversity on the BDNF gene. Biol Psychiatry 2009;65(9):760–9.

56. Calabrese F, Molteni R, Racagni G, et al. Neuronal plasticity: a link between stress and mood disorders. Psychoneuroendocrinology 2009;34(Suppl 1):S208–16.

57. McGowan PO, Sasaki A, D'Alessio AC, et al. Epigenetic regulation of the glucocorticoid receptor in human brain associates with childhood abuse. Nat Neurosci 2009;12(3):342–8.

58. Bugental DB, Happaney K. Predicting infant maltreatment in low-income families: the interactive effects of maternal attributions and child status at birth. Dev Psychol 2004;40(2):234–43.

59. Spencer N, Wallace A, Sundrum R, et al. Child abuse registration, fetal growth, and preterm birth: a population based study. J Epidemiol Community Health 2006;60(4):337–40.

60. Sullivan RM, Shokrai N, Leon M. Physical stimulation reduces the body temperature of infant rats. Dev Psychobiol 1988;21(3):225–35.

61. Champagne FA, Meaney MJ. Stress during gestation alters postpartum maternal care and the development of the offspring in a rodent model. Biol Psychiatry 2006;59(12):1227–35.

62. Kaplan LA, Evans L, Monk C. Effects of mothers' prenatal psychiatric status and postnatal caregiving on infant biobehavioral regulation: can prenatal programming be modified? Early Hum Dev 2008;84(4):249–56.
63. McLaughlin KA, Zeanah CH, Fox NA, et al. Attachment security as a mechanism linking foster care placement to improved mental health outcomes in previously institutionalized children. J Child Psychol Psychiatry 2011. [Epub ahead of print].
64. Fox NA, Almas AN, Degnan KA, et al. The effects of severe psychosocial deprivation and foster care intervention on cognitive development at 8 years of age: findings from the Bucharest Early Intervention Project. J Child Psychol Psychiatry 2011;52(9):919–28.
65. Champagne FA, Meaney MJ. Transgenerational effects of social environment on variations in maternal care and behavioral response to novelty. Behav Neurosci 2007;121(6):1353–63.
66. Francis DD, Diorio J, Plotsky PM, et al. Environmental enrichment reverses the effects of maternal separation on stress reactivity. J Neurosci 2002;22(18): 7840–3.
67. Morley-Fletcher S, Rea M, Maccari S, et al. Environmental enrichment during adolescence reverses the effects of prenatal stress on play behaviour and HPA axis reactivity in rats. Eur J Neurosci 2003;18(12):3367–74.
68. Weaver IC, Champagne FA, Brown SE, et al. Reversal of maternal programming of stress responses in adult offspring through methyl supplementation: altering epigenetic marking later in life. J Neurosci 2005;25(47):11045–54.
69. Jirtle RL, Skinner MK. Environmental epigenomics and disease susceptibility. Nat Rev Genet 2007;8(4):253–62.
70. Franklin TB, Russig H, Weiss IC, et al. Epigenetic transmission of the impact of early stress across generations. Biol Psychiatry 2010;68(5):408–15.
71. Champagne FA. Epigenetic mechanisms and the transgenerational effects of maternal care. Front Neuroendocrinol 2008;29(3):386–97.
72. Devlin AM, Brain U, Austin J, et al. Prenatal exposure to maternal depressed mood and the MTHFR C677T variant affect SLC6A4 methylation in infants at birth. PLoS One 2010;5(8):e12201.
73. van IJzendoorn MH, Caspers K, Bakermans-Kranenburg MJ, et al. Methylation matters: interaction between methylation density and serotonin transporter genotype predicts unresolved loss or trauma. Biol Psychiatry 2010;68(5):405–7.

Developmental Care for High-Risk Newborns: Emerging Science, Clinical Application, and Continuity from Newborn Intensive Care Unit to Community

Joy V. Browne, PhD, PCNS-BC[a,b,*]

KEYWORDS

- High-risk neonate • Developmental care • Infant development
- Attachment • Kangaroo mother care

NEURODEVELOPMENTAL OUTCOMES OF HIGH-RISK NEWBORNS

Neonatology has made astounding technological, pharmacologic, and intervention changes over the last 4 decades, resulting in the survival of earlier-born and sicker infants worldwide. However, the prevalence of major sensory and more subtle cognitive, communication, motor, and neurodevelopmental sequelae, both short and long term, have not shown concomitant improvement, particularly in the very-low–birth weight and extremely low–birth weight categories.[1–3] In addition, more attention has been

---

Funding for this article is in part from the US Department of Health and Human Services, Administration on Developmental Disabilities, University Center of Excellence in Developmental Disabilities Education, Research, and Service grant number 90DD0632 and the Maternal and Child Health Bureau, Leadership Education in Neurodevelopmental Disabilities (LEND) grant number T73-MC11044.
[a] JFK Partners Center for Family and Infant Interaction, University of Colorado Anschutz Medical Campus, 13121 East 19th Avenue, L-28 Room 5117, Aurora, CO, USA
[b] School of Nursing and Midwifery, Queen's University of Belfast, Belfast, Northern Ireland
* JFK Partners Center for Family and Infant Interaction, University of Colorado Anschutz Medical Campus, 13121 East 19th Avenue, L-28 Room 5117, Aurora, CO.
E-mail address: Joy.Browne@childrenscolorado.org

Clin Perinatol 38 (2011) 719–729
doi:10.1016/j.clp.2011.08.003

directed to the identification of preterm and low–birth weight infants who also develop mental health issues such as attention-deficit and attention-deficit/hyperactivity disorders, anxiety disorders, and difficulties with emotion regulation.[4–10] Many investigators have identified a significant proportion of prematurely born children as having behaviors consistent with a diagnosis of autistic disorder.[11–13] In addition, recent findings of a large cohort of infants in Europe showed that infants with lower gestational ages showed crying, eating and sleeping problems, indicative of early regulatory disorders.[14,15] The occurrence of 1 or more of these regulatory difficulties in the first few months of life were found to be predictive of later cognitive and behavioral challenges as they increased into the toddler and preschool years.[16]

The cause of these findings is not readily understood, but it is thought that early environmental influences on the brain during a particularly sensitive developmental period account for some of these nonoptimal neurodevelopmental outcomes. To date, no specific pharmacologic or technologic strategies have been offered to ameliorate these findings.

EMERGENCE OF DEVELOPMENTAL CARE

The practice of developmentally supportive care (DSC) has evolved over the recent decades, with variations in definition and clinical application but an overarching primary goal of improving the short- and long-term neurodevelopmental outcomes of high-risk newborns. Early recognition of the physiologic impact of the acoustic environment and handling on the high-risk newborn prompted investigations of how professionals might modify the caregiving environment in the newborn intensive care unit (NICU) to reduce stress and promote development.[17,18] Professionals began to understand the detrimental impact of overwhelming sensory input and procedures on the developing newborn brain[19,20] and proposed the term environmental neonatology[21] to address this emerging science. Simultaneously, the unique behavioral organization of the high-risk newborn was being described[22–25] and advances in knowledge of the effect of stressful environments on brain development were being articulated.[26] As professionals recognized the potential to reduce or modify the impact of the physical and caregiving environment on infant neurodevelopment, approaches described as DSC and neurodevelopmental therapy were introduced into the vocabulary and practice of NICU professionals.[20,27,28] Early interdisciplinary study panels that synthesized the then current thinking regarding both the sensory as well as the caregiving environment for high-risk newborns provided a blueprint for further research necessary for a scientific foundation to improve the physical approaches and articulates developmental care approaches. The field became recognized as having empirically evaluated interventions and recommendations for interventions.[29,30] An emphasis was also put on the incorporation of more humane caregiving for high-risk infants and their parents.[31,32]

Further research into the impact of the caregiving environment revealed significant physiologic and behavioral disorganization responses to obviously painful and stressful procedures.[33–36] The experience of repeated pain by the neonate can have significant short- and long-term consequences for brain organization during sensitive periods of development.[37–39] Infant responses to being handled and to typical NICU caregiving routines and procedures such as bathing,[40,41] weighing,[42,43] and diaper change[44–46] indicated that these seemingly innocuous events were also perceived as stressful to the developing infant. Although a review of pain amelioration is not addressed in this article, the reduction of painful procedures and the support of the infant during necessary noxious procedures is a priority of developmentally supportive caregiving.

EMERGING CONTRIBUTIONS OF BASIC SCIENCE TO UNDERSTANDING EARLY DEVELOPMENT

As clinical studies of DSC were developing in NICUs, developmental psychobiologists were providing an understanding of early development from a basic science perspective. Because of the differences in foci and application of basic science and clinical research, few of their studies were applied to understanding the developing human newborn. However, the contributions of these psychobiologists in the areas of sensory development, chemosensory recognition, tactile and kinesthetic development, epigenetic consequences of early birth, and the role of the early parent-infant attachment relationship (see reviews by Sullivan and colleagues; Champagne and colleagues elsewhere in this issue) have assisted NICU professionals in the application of basic science findings to clinical questions that cannot be examined in the human neonate. Their work has emphasized the potential for sensitive periods in fetal and newborn brain development. These psychobiologists have articulated the importance of experience-dependent and experience-expectant development and have contributed to our understanding of environmental influences on brain organization. They have also assisted us in the understanding of the importance of the early attachment relationship between the offspring's mother, based on unique sensory, thermoregulatory, and circadian rhythm cues (for application of these findings to NICU care[47–49]).

EMERGENCE OF ENVIRONMENTAL DESIGN CHANGES

The environment in which newborns live and grow influences their development and is an integral contributor to how developmental care is provided. The physical environment, including light, sound, temperature, activity, and space has an impact on development, just as the caregiving environment has an impact. Recognizing the emerging science of healing environments and their contribution to optimal health outcomes, interdisciplinary consensus panels for NICU design have developed evidence-based standards for developmentally supportive environments.[29,30] Provision of optimal developmental care requires sufficient environmental modification for infants to have ready access to their familiar and unique mothers (and fathers) who are able to provide a consistent, intimate, regulatory secure base for development. Incorporated into the NICU design standards are recommendations for enough space, supports, and considerations for restful, private, and nurturing caregiving by the baby's family. Single family room design is now emerging as the optimal environment for neonates and their family[29,50] (also see article by White elsewhere in this issue).

The caregiving environment for newborns is ideally provided by the mother's body. For several decades kangaroo mother care, otherwise known as skin-to-skin care, has been used to provide an early regulatory and nurturing experience for newborns. Recent research has provided ample data on the safety and efficacy of this approach even with high-risk newborns.[51–53] A combination of a family-centered environment, individualized developmental care, and almost exclusive kangaroo mother care in a Swedish NICU has demonstrated a significant reduction in length of hospitalization.[52] Promoting the family's presence for the entire length of stay could be the catalyst of this synergistic approach to NICU developmental caregiving and could result in more competent parenting over the continuum of the first days, weeks, and months of the infant's life.

DSC IN THE NICU

The term developmental care is frequently associated with the work of Heidelise Als, a pioneer in neurodevelopmental assessment and intervention for preterm infants.

Als and colleagues have provided the most theoretically driven, systematically applied, and rigorously evaluated developmental care approach to date. Described as individualized DSC, their approach incorporates regularly scheduled observations of the individual infant's behavioral communication before, during, and after a caregiving intervention and, using those observations, summarizes the infant's developmental goals and provides recommendations for caregiving (for a comprehensive description, go to www.nidcap.org). The Newborn Individualized Developmental Care and Assessment Program (NIDCAP) provides comprehensive and in-depth training in this approach.[54] Elements of NIDCAP address modification of the sensory environment, including the bed space and bedding; being responsive to the infant's communicated strengths, needs, and goals; and integration of the parent into the intimate care of the infant. Throughout the training and application of the approach, emphasis is on supporting a nurturing and growth-promoting relationship between caregivers and infants, professionals, and family members as well as among professionals.

Als and colleagues[55–57] have demonstrated comprehensive research into the application and outcomes of the NIDCAP work. NIDCAP studies have shown advantageous medical, neurobehavioral, and brain structure and function effects for very-low–birth weight infants in the newborn period[58–61] and consistency into adolescence.[62,63] Buehler[64] showed neurodevelopmental benefits for a later-born and higher weight group of infants using the NIDCAP approach. More recently, Als and colleagues[65] demonstrated that brain structure and function as well as behavioral organization in intrauterine growth-restricted infants were enhanced after application of the NIDCAP.

Other investigators have replicated the NIDCAP approach in larger populations of infants than were included in Als and colleagues' original studies. Peters and colleagues[66] found that length of hospitalization and incidence of chronic lung disease was reduced in NIDCAP-treated infants and, at 18 months' corrected age, the children were less likely to have a disability. However, in another large study, Maguire and colleagues[67] did not find similar beneficial results of NIDCAP. The question of a dose response has been offered because the infants in this study were transferred to outlying hospitals much more quickly than in other related research and may not have had repeated NIDCAP observations and ongoing intervention. Considerable interest has been generated regarding the NIDCAP individualized developmental care approach, prompting several comprehensive reviews of research findings.[68–70] All reviews call for more research of individualized developmental care that can address limitations in the current studies and determine factors that have led to a variety of positive short-term outcomes. Regardless of the acceptance of the benefits of NIDCAP from a scientific perspective, in clinical practice there have been no detrimental effects noted by the application of this approach in NICUs. Instead, the infusion of the NIDCAP work into NICU caregiving practices is experiencing global implementation.

THE EARLY INTERVENTION CONTINUUM

DSC could be perceived to be on a continuum of early intervention that starts with good prenatal care, including attention to the mother's physical and mental health and continues throughout the hospital NICU stay and then after the infant has been discharged to the community. James Heckman,[71] a Nobel laureate in economics, has postulated that investment in early intervention can produce long-term benefits to not only the individual and the family but also the society. His recent antenatal investment hypothesis proposes an economic rationale for intervention even to the antenatal period to have the best personal, social, and government economic return.[72]

Results of a variety of early intervention studies have cumulatively documented the importance of nurturing and responsive relationships between children and their primary caregivers[73] and have resulted in children whose socioemotional development is supportive of optimal cognitive development and behavioral regulation. An increasing number of early intervention studies for high-risk infants have provided a continuum of developmental care from NICU to home. Rauh and colleagues[74] developed the Mother-Infant Transaction Program (MITP), which provided mothers of high-risk very-low–birth weight newborns guidance in interacting with their infants during 7 one-hour sessions in the NICU and then 4 home visits during the infant's early months. These guidance sessions were similar in basic concepts to the individualized developmental care strategies used in NIDCAP programs and based on the support of the ongoing mother-infant dyadic relationship. Seven- and 9-year outcomes revealed significantly higher achievement scores and general cognitive outcomes favoring the infants who received the intervention compared with those who did not.[75,76] Recently, several European and Australian early intervention programs have adapted the MITP approach to their settings and have demonstrated more optimal parent-infant interactions,[77] cognitive scores at 5 years,[78] behavioral and brain organization, and a reduction of parent stress.[79–81] Other early intervention programs not started until after discharge have also shown positive effects on achievement scores and behavior. The Infant Behavior Assessment and Intervention Program, adapted from the NIDCAP approach in the NICU,[82] has shown motor improvements at 24 months.[83] Other studies that have focused on the mother-infant relationship have described less maternal depression and anxiety in the mothers after intervention, likely influencing not only the relationship but also infant developmental outcome.[58,82] Of note is a report on the 18-year follow-up of the Infant Health and Behavior Project, which provided intensive home- and center-based intervention after discharge from the NICU; this study found more optimal achievement outcomes for higher–birth weight children than those born at a lower birth weight.[84] Taken together, these developmentally supportive early intervention approaches may prove to have positive effects on the mother-infant relationship, behavioral regulation, and later cognitive and motor function.

Intervention for high-risk newborns has typically been segmented into either NICU developmental care or home- or center-based early intervention services. It may be that providing a continuum of care, using similar theoretical foundations and intervention strategies that focus on early parent-infant relationships, will prove to provide neuroprotection in the respective caregiving environments. It is well known that children in families who experience multiple social and economic risk factors suffer cognitively and behaviorally when compared with children whose families do not experience similar risks.[85] Provision of developmentally appropriate, family supportive, early intervention begins with excellent prenatal preparation for parenting and prevention of early birth. Sensitive individualized DSC provided in the NICU should also support the competent parenting through enhanced parent-infant relationship and continue throughout the early months after discharge. This provision of a continuum of care may provide the answers to the questions regarding possible benefits for optimizing infant neurodevelopmental outcomes.[86] It is essential for NICU professionals to ensure collaboration with community resources, evaluation of infants for the development of their Individual Family Service Plan, and follow-up with the community early intervention team.[87,88]

ASSESSMENT OF NEURODEVELOPMENTAL OUTCOMES

Most neurodevelopmental outcome studies focus primarily on cognitive, communication, and motor functioning. However, many of the neurobehavioral evaluation instruments used perinatally are not reliably predictive of later outcomes,[89] may not be sensitive enough to distinguish more subtle developmental deficits,[89,90] or do not assess early regulation as a contributing factor in the infant's development. Longer-term outcomes of developmentally supportive intervention provided in the NICU, perhaps more subtle than are currently measured by typical outcome measures, may not be distinguishable with currently used evaluation instruments. Current research that provides more sensitive and rigorously evaluated early assessments is beginning to predict later outcomes.[89,91] Redefining what outcome or outcomes may reflect optimal neurodevelopment and resulting brain organization may help the field to determine the most appropriate developmentally supportive intervention that is needed. For example, better techniques of determining the impact of early regulatory disorders of feeding, crying, and sleeping along with appropriate evidence-based intervention programs may not only enhance the infant's organization during a potentially sensitive period of brain development but also affect the caregiving relationship between the infant and the mother.

SUMMARY

Neonatology has invested much in technological, pharmacologic, and medical intervention strategies which have improved the survival of increasingly younger and sicker newborns. However, improving neurodevelopmental and socioemotional outcomes has been elusive. DSC aims to ameliorate these potential consequences and contribute to better brain organization during periods of rapid growth and development. DSC for high-risk newborns focuses on understanding the baby's communicated developmental goals and supporting his or her attempts to become organized at a higher level of development. It also respects and advocates for the mother's (and father's) availability to be the infant's best regulator, comforter, nurturer, and protector. Developmental care is informed by and integrates knowledge from basic developmental science, contributions of environmental design, the sensory impact on brain development, and clinical studies of the effect of NICU caregiving on infant organization. Individualized developmentally supportive caregiving provided by the NIDCAP approach is the most rigorously studied and organized program to support relationship-based intervention. More extensive and thorough research needs to be conducted to determine the specifics of benefits and risks of optimizing infant neurodevelopmental outcomes. It seems prudent to provide similarly designed and theoretically similar approaches across NICUs and home intervention for continuity and family support.

REFERENCES

1. Hack M, Taylor HG, Drotar D, et al. Chronic conditions, functional limitations, and special health care needs of school-aged children born with extremely low-birth-weight in the 1990s. JAMA 2005;294(3):318–25.
2. Hack M. Survival and neurodevelopmental outcomes of preterm infants. J Pediatr Gastroenterol Nutr 2007;45(Suppl 3):S141–2.
3. Wilson-Costello D, Friedman H, Minich N, et al. Improved survival rates with increased neurodevelopmental disability for extremely low birth weight infants in the 1990s. Pediatrics 2005;115(4):997–1003.

4. Vanderbilt D, Gleason MM. Mental health concerns of the premature infant through the lifespan. Child Adolesc Psychiatr Clin N Am 2010;19(2):211–28, vii–viii.
5. Johnson S, Hollis C, Kochhar P, et al. Psychiatric disorders in extremely preterm children: longitudinal finding at age 11 years in the EPICure study. J Am Acad Child Adolesc Psychiatry 2010;49(5):453–63, e451.
6. Hack M, Taylor HG, Schluchter M, et al. Behavioral outcomes of extremely low birth weight children at age 8 years. J Dev Behav Pediatr 2009;30(2):122–30.
7. Delobel-Ayoub M, Arnaud C, White-Koning M, et al. Behavioral problems and cognitive performance at 5 years of age after very preterm birth: the EPIPAGE Study. Pediatrics 2009;123(6):1485–92.
8. van Baar AL, Vermaas J, Knots E, et al. Functioning at school age of moderately preterm children born at 32 to 36 weeks' gestational age. Pediatrics 2009;124(1): 251–7.
9. Heinonen K, Raikkonen K, Pesonen AK, et al. Behavioural symptoms of attention deficit/hyperactivity disorder in preterm and term children born small and appropriate for gestational age: a longitudinal study. BMC Pediatr 2010;10:91.
10. Hille ET, den Ouden AL, Saigal S, et al. Behavioural problems in children who weigh 1000 g or less at birth in four countries. Lancet 2001;357(9269): 1641–3.
11. Kuban KC, O'Shea TM, Allred EN, et al. Positive screening on the Modified Checklist for Autism in Toddlers (M-CHAT) in extremely low gestational age newborns. J Pediatr 2009;154(4):535–40, e531.
12. Limperopoulos C. Extreme prematurity, cerebellar injury, and autism. Semin Pediatr Neurol 2010;17(1):25–9.
13. Limperopoulos C. Autism spectrum disorders in survivors of extreme prematurity. Clin Perinatol 2009;36(4):791–805, vi.
14. Schmid G, Schreier A, Meyer R, et al. A prospective study on the persistence of infant crying, sleeping and feeding problems and preschool behaviour. Acta Paediatr 2010;99(2):286–90.
15. Wolke D, Schmid G, Schreier A, et al. Crying and feeding problems in infancy and cognitive outcome in preschool children born at risk: a prospective population study. J Dev Behav Pediatr 2009;30(3):226–38.
16. Hemmi MH, Wolke D, Schneider S. Associations between problems with crying, sleeping and/or feeding in infancy and long-term behavioural outcomes in childhood: a meta-analysis. Arch Dis Child 2011;96(7):622–9.
17. Long JG, Lucey JF, Philip AG. Noise and hypoxemia in the intensive care nursery. Pediatrics 1980;65(1):143–5.
18. Long JG, Philip AG, Lucey JF. Excessive handling as a cause of hypoxemia. Pediatrics 1980;65(2):203–7.
19. Gorski PA, Hole WT, Leonard CH, et al. Direct computer recording of premature infants and nursery care: distress following two interventions. Pediatrics 1983; 72(2):198–202.
20. Gorski PA, Lewkowicz DJ, Huntington L, et al. Early neurodevelopmental therapy. Lancet 1986;1(8478):444–5.
21. Gottfried AW, Hodgman JE, Brown KW. How intensive is newborn intensive care? An environmental analysis. Pediatrics 1984;74(2):292–4.
22. Gorski PA, Davison MF, Brazelton TB. Stages of behavioral organization in the high-risk neonate: theoretical and clinical considerations. Semin Perinatol 1979; 3(1):61–72.
23. Als H. The newborn communicates. J Commun 1977;27(2):66–73.

24. Als H, Brazelton TB. A new model of assessing the behavioral organization in preterm and fullterm infants: two case studies. J Am Acad Child Psychiatry 1981;20(2):239–63.
25. Als H, Duffy FH. Neurobehavioral assessment in the newborn period: opportunity for early detection of later learning disabilities and for early intervention. Birth Defects Orig Artic Ser 1989;25(6):127–52.
26. Nelson CA, Carver LJ. The effects of stress and trauma on brain and memory: a view from developmental cognitive neuroscience. Dev Psychopathol 1998; 10(4):793–809.
27. Als H, Gilkerson L. The role of relationship-based developmentally supportive newborn intensive care in strengthening outcome of preterm infants. Semin Perinatol 1997;21(3):178–89.
28. Goodman M, Rothberg AD, Houston-McMillan JE, et al. Effect of early neurodevelopmental therapy in normal and at-risk survivors of neonatal intensive care. Lancet 1985;2:1327–30.
29. White RD. The newborn intensive care unit environment of care: how we got here, where we're headed, and why. Semin Perinatol 2011;35(1):2–7.
30. White RD. Recommended standards for the newborn ICU. J Perinatol 2007; 27(Suppl 2):S4–19.
31. Sizun J, Ratynski N, Boussard C. Humane neonatal care initiative, NIDCAP and family-centred neonatal intensive care. Neonatal Individualized Developmental Care and Assessment Program. Acta Paediatr 1999;88(10):1172.
32. Levin A. Humane neonatal care initiative. Acta Paediatr 1999;88(4):353–5.
33. Anand KJ. Effects of perinatal pain and stress. Prog Brain Res 2000;122:117–29.
34. Holsti L, Grunau RE. Extremity movements help occupational therapists identify stress responses in preterm infants in the neonatal intensive care unit: a systematic review. Can J Occup Ther 2007;74(3):183–94.
35. Gressens P, Rogido M, Paindaveine B, et al. The impact of neonatal intensive care practices on the developing brain. J Pediatr 2002;140(6):646–53.
36. Grunau RE, Holsti L, Whitfield MF, et al. Are twitches, startles, and body movements pain indicators in extremely low birth weight infants? Clin J Pain 2000; 16(1):37–45.
37. Anand KJ. Pain, plasticity, and premature birth: a prescription for permanent suffering? Nat Med 2000;6(9):971–3.
38. Grunau RE, Tu MT, Whitfield MF, et al. Cortisol, behavior, and heart rate reactivity to immunization pain at 4 months corrected age in infants born very preterm. Clin J Pain 2010;26(8):698–704.
39. Bhutta AT, Anand KJ. Vulnerability of the developing brain. Neuronal mechanisms. Clin Perinatol 2002;29(3):357–72.
40. Peters KL. Bathing premature infants: physiological and behavioral consequences. Am J Crit Care 1998;7(2):90–100.
41. Liaw JJ, Yang L, Chang LH, et al. Improving neonatal caregiving through a developmentally supportive care training program. Appl Nurs Res 2009;22(2):86–93.
42. Catelin C, Tordjman S, Morin V, et al. Clinical, physiologic, and biologic impact of environmental and behavioral interventions in neonates during a routine nursing procedure. J Pain 2005;6(12):791–7.
43. Neu M, Browne JV. Infant physiologic and behavioral organization during swaddled versus unswaddled weighing. J Perinatol 1997;17(3):193–8.
44. Perry EH, Bada HS, Ray JD, et al. Blood pressure increases, birth weight-dependent stability boundary, and intraventricular hemorrhage. Pediatrics 1990;85(5):727.

45. Limperopoulos C, Gauvreau KK, O'Leary H, et al. Cerebral hemodynamic changes during intensive care of preterm infants. Pediatrics 2008;122(5): e1006–13.

46. Mörelius E, Hellström-Westas L, Carlén C, et al. Is a nappy change stressful to neonates? Early Hum Dev 2006;82(10):669–76.

47. Graven SN, Browne J. Sensory development in the fetus, neonate, and infant: introduction and overview. Newborn Infant Nurs Rev 2008;8(4):169–72.

48. Graven S. Sleep and brain development. Clin Perinatol 2006;33(3):693–706, vii.

49. Browne J, Graven SN, Browne J. Chemosensory development of the fetus and newborn. Newborn Infant Nurs Rev 2008;8(4):180–6.

50. Lester BM, Miller RJ, Hawes K, et al. Infant neurobehavioral development. Semin Perinatol 2011;35(1):8–19.

51. Nyqvist KH, Anderson GC, Bergman N, et al. State of the art and recommendations. Kangaroo mother care: application in a high-tech environment. Acta Paediatr 2010;99(6):812–9.

52. Ortenstrand A, Westrup B, Brostrom EB, et al. The Stockholm Neonatal Family Centered Care Study: effects on length of stay and infant morbidity. Pediatrics 2010;125(2):e278–85.

53. Browne JV. Early relationship environments: physiology of skin-to-skin contact for parents and their preterm infants. Clin Perinatol 2004;31(2):287–98, vii.

54. Lawhon G, Hedlund RE. Newborn individualized developmental care and assessment program training and education. J Perinat Neonatal Nurs 2008; 22(2):133–44 [quiz: 145–6].

55. Als H, Lawhon G, Duffy FH, et al. Individualized developmental care for the very low-birth-weight preterm infant. Medical and neurofunctional effects [see comment]. JAMA 1994;272:853–8.

56. Als H, Duffy FH, McAnulty GB. Effectiveness of individualized neurodevelopmental care in the newborn intensive care unit (NICU). Acta Paediatr Suppl 1996;416:21–30.

57. Als H, Duffy FH, McAnulty GB, et al. Early experience alters brain function and structure. Pediatrics 2004;113:846–57.

58. Kleberg A, Westrup B, Stjernqvist K. Developmental outcome, child behaviour and mother-child interaction at 3 years of age following Newborn Individualized Developmental Care and Intervention Program (NIDCAP) intervention. Early Hum Dev 2000;60(2):123–35.

59. Westrup B, Bohm B, Lagercrantz H, et al. Preschool outcome in children born very prematurely and cared for according to the Newborn Individualized Developmental Care and Assessment Program (NIDCAP). Acta Paediatr 2004;93(4): 498–507.

60. Westrup B, Stjernqvist K, Kleberg A, et al. Neonatal individualized care in practice: a Swedish experience. Semin Neonatol 2002;7(6):447–57.

61. Fleisher BE, VandenBerg K, Constantinou J, et al. Individualized developmental care for very-low-birth-weight premature infants. Clin Pediatr (Phila) 1995;34(10):523–9.

62. McAnulty GB, Duffy FH, Butler SC, et al. Effects of the Newborn Individualized Developmental Care and Assessment Program (NIDCAP) at age 8 years: preliminary data. Clin Pediatr (Phila) 2010;49(3):258–70.

63. McAnulty G, Duffy FH, Butler S, et al. Individualized developmental care for a large sample of very preterm infants: health, neurobehaviour and neurophysiology. Acta Paediatr 2009;98(12):1920–6.

64. Buehler DM, Als H, Duffy FH, et al. Effectiveness of individualized developmental care for low-risk preterm infants: behavioral and electrophysiologic evidence. Pediatrics 1995;96(5 Pt 1):923–32.

65. Als H, Duffy FH, McAnulty GB, et al. Is the Newborn Individualized Developmental Care and Assessment Program (NIDCAP) effective for preterm infants with intrauterine growth restriction? J Perinatol 2011;31(2):130–6.
66. Peters KL, Rosychuk RJ, Hendson L, et al. Improvement of short- and long-term outcomes for very low birth weight infants: Edmonton NIDCAP trial. Pediatrics 2009;124(4):1009–20.
67. Maguire CM, Walther FJ, Sprij AJ, et al. Effects of individualized developmental care in a randomized trial of preterm infants <32 weeks. Pediatrics 2009; 124(4):1021–30.
68. Symington A, Pinelli J. Developmental care for promoting development and preventing morbidity in preterm infants. Cochrane Database Syst Rev 2006;2:CD001814.
69. Wallin L, Eriksson M. Newborn Individual Development Care and Assessment Program (NIDCAP): a systematic review of the literature. Worldviews Evid Based Nurs 2009;6(2):54–69.
70. Legendre V, Burtner PA, Martinez KL, et al. The evolving practice of developmental care in the neonatal unit: a systematic review. Phys Occup Ther Pediatr 2011;31(3):315–38.
71. Heckman JJ. Schools, skills, and synapses. Econ Inq 2008;46(3):289–324.
72. Doyle O, Harmon CP, Heckman JJ, et al. Investing in early human development: timing and economic efficiency. Econ Hum Biol 2009;7(1):1–6.
73. Shonkoff JP, Phillips D, Board on Children Youth and Families (U.S.), Committee on Integrating the Science of Early Childhood Development. From neurons to neighborhoods: the science of early childhood development. Washington, DC: National Academy Press; 2000.
74. Rauh VA, Nurcombe B, Achenbach T, et al. The Mother-Infant Transaction Program. The content and implications of an intervention for the mothers of low-birthweight infants. Clin Perinatol 1990;17(1):31–45.
75. Achenbach TM, Howell CT, Aoki MF, et al. Nine-year outcome of the Vermont intervention program for low birth weight infants. Pediatrics 1993;91(1):45–55.
76. Achenbach TM, Phares V, Howell CT, et al. Seven-year outcome of the Vermont Intervention Program for Low-Birthweight Infants. Child Dev 1990;61(6):1672–81.
77. Ravn IH, Smith L, Lindemann R, et al. Effect of early intervention on social interaction between mothers and preterm infants at 12 months of age: a randomized controlled trial. Infant Behav Dev 2011;34(2):215–25.
78. Nordhov SM, Rånning JA, Dahl LB, et al. Early intervention improves cognitive outcomes for preterm infants: randomized controlled trial. Pediatrics 2010; 126(5):e1088–94.
79. Kaaresen PI, Rønning JA, Tunby J, et al. A randomized controlled trial of an early intervention program in low birth weight children: outcome at 2 years. Early Hum Dev 2008;84(3):201–9.
80. Newnham CA, Milgrom J, Skouteris H. Effectiveness of a modified Mother-Infant Transaction Program on outcomes for preterm infants from 3 to 24 months of age. Infant Behav Dev 2009;32(1):17–26.
81. Milgrom J, Newnham C, Anderson PJ, et al. Early sensitivity training for parents of preterm infants: impact on the developing brain. Pediatr Res 2010;67(3):330–5.
82. Spittle AJ, Anderson PJ, Lee KJ, et al. Preventive care at home for very preterm infants improves infant and caregiver outcomes at 2 years. Pediatrics 2010; 126(1):e171–8.
83. Koldewijn K, van Wassenaer A, Wolf MJ, et al. A neurobehavioral intervention and assessment program in very low birth weight infants: outcome at 24 months. J Pediatr 2010;156(3):359–65.

84. McCormick MC, Brooks-Gunn J, Buka SL, et al. Early intervention in low birth weight premature infants: results at 18 years of age for the Infant Health and Development Program. Pediatrics 2006;117:771–80.

85. Sameroff AJ. Environmental risk factors in infancy. Pediatrics 1998;102(5 Suppl E): 1287–92.

86. Browne JV, Talmi A. Family-based intervention to enhance infant-parent relationships in the neonatal intensive care unit. J Pediatr Psychol 2005;30(8):667–77.

87. Bondurant PG, Brinkman KS. Developmentally supportive care in the newborn intensive care unit: early intervention in the community. Nurs Clin North Am 2003;38(2):253–69.

88. Browne JV, Langlois A, Ross ES, et al. Beginnings: an interim individualized family service plan for use in the intensive care nursery. Infants Young Child 2001;14(2): 19–32.

89. El-Dib M, Massaro AN, Glass P, et al. Neurodevelopmental assessment of the newborn: an opportunity for prediction of outcome. Brain Dev 2011;33(2):95–105.

90. Heineman KR, Hadders-Algra M. Evaluation of neuromotor function in infancy—a systematic review of available methods. Jnbsp;Dev Behav Pediatr 2008;29(4): 315–23.

91. Liu J, Bann C, Lester B, et al. Neonatal neurobehavior predicts medical and behavioral outcome. Pediatrics 2010;125(1):e90–8.

Eating as a Neurodevelopmental Process for High-Risk Newborns

Joy V. Browne, PhD, PCNS-BC[a,b,*], Erin Sundseth Ross, PhD, CCC-SLP[a]

KEYWORDS

- High-risk neonate • Infant feeding behaviors
- Infant development • Attachment • Infant growth

FEEDING DISORDERS IN THE HIGH-RISK INFANT

Discharge of the high-risk newborn from the neonatal intensive care unit (NICU) typically includes successful volume and rate of oral intake by either breast or bottle, and appropriate and consistent weight gain for specified amounts of time.[1] Delay in discharge is often attributed to a lack of attaining success at eating skills and adequate growth. These delays often cause frustration for the parents who are anxious to have their baby home, and frustration for the professional staff, including the case manager, who are also anxious to save hospitalization costs and lengthy stays.

Feeding problems develop through interactions among biological, behavioral, and environmental factors, and preterm infants and their families, especially infants born extremely preterm, are at high risk for feeding problems, developmental delay, and relationship difficulties as well as compromised growth.[2–4] Adequate growth is typically regarded as a positive outcome for high-risk infants but is difficult to achieve in the NICU. The majority of growth faltering occurs in the initial hospitalization for a myriad of infant and medical reasons, including nutrient absorption and gut

Preparation of this article was supported in part by grant from the Maternal and Child Health Bureau. Funding for this article is in part from the US Department of Health and Human Services, Administration on Developmental Disabilities, University Center of Excellence in Developmental Disabilities Education, Research, and Service Grant #90DD0632 and the Maternal and Child Health Bureau, Leadership Education in Neurodevelopmental Disabilities (LEND) Grant # T73-MC11044.
J.V.B. has nothing to disclose; E.S.R. is a consultant for Nestle/Gerber.
[a] JFK Partners Center for Family and Infant Interaction, University of Colorado Anschutz Medical Campus, L-28 Room 5117, 13121 East 19th Avenue, Aurora, CO 80045, USA
[b] School of Nursing and Midwifery, Queen's University of Belfast, Belfast, Northern Ireland
* Corresponding author. JFK Partners Center for Family and Infant Interaction, University of Colorado Anschutz Medical Campus, L-28 Room 5117, 13121 East 19th Avenue, Aurora, CO 80045.
E-mail address: Joy.Browne@childrenscolorado.org

Clin Perinatol 38 (2011) 731–743
doi:10.1016/j.clp.2011.08.004
0095-5108/11/$ – see front matter © 2011 Elsevier Inc. All rights reserved.

intolerance.[5] Much attention has been focused on the need for improved growth in the initial hospital stay, as the highest rate of growth has been correlated with both a reduced risk of developmental delay and better growth at 18 months corrected age.[6]

Early weight gain is known to be predictive of later growth in term infants, and is likely predictive in the preterm population as well. Ross and colleagues[7] found that term infants who lost a significant amount of weight between their 4- and 6-month well child visits were more likely to have growth faltering when compared with those whose weight for age did not shift as significantly. As low birth weight (LBW) and very low birth weight (VLBW) infants transition to home, in the short term they are likely to have poorer weight gain than their larger counterparts. Deloian[8] found that LBW infants gained an average of 35 g per day and VLBW infants gained only 18.7 g per day. Ross[9] examined preterm infants both at term and 2 weeks corrected age. Weight gain per day between term and 2 weeks ranged from 6.3 to 90.3 g per day, indicating great variability in infant growth. After discharge from the NICU many high-risk infants experience growth faltering.[7] Dusick and colleagues,[10] as part of the National Institute of Child Health and Human Development Neonatal Research Network, evaluated infants within 14 centers for growth problems. At 36 weeks gestational age, 97% of VLBW infants weighed less than the 10th percentile for their age, and of those with birth weights of 501 to 1000 g, 99% had weights less than the 10th percentile. At 18 to 22 months corrected age, 40% of these infants continued to have weight, length, and head circumferences less than the 10th percentile.

Wood and colleagues5 studied infants born at less than 26 weeks' gestation who were AGA, and found weight and head circumference z-scores that fell below the mean at both the estimated due date and at 30 months corrected age. Dodrill and colleagues[10,11] found the mean lengths and weights of preterm, AGA Australian infants were significantly less than their term counterparts across all time points (term, 4 months, 8 months, and 12 months corrected age). Those infants born small for gestational age (SGA) had greater weight faltering (defined as a weight for age less than the 10th percentile) than did those born average for gestational age (AGA), 69% and 42%, respectively.[10]

Feeding problems are even more prevalent than are growth problems in the preterm population. Hawdon and colleagues[12] followed 35 infants with a mean gestational age of 34 weeks at birth, and found 40% of them with poor coordination of sucking, swallowing, and breathing at the time of assessment in the NICU (between 36 and 40 weeks postmenstrual age). At 6 months, these same infants who had poor coordination continued to demonstrate increased feeding difficulties. These infants were 6 times more likely to vomit and 3 times more likely to cough during mealtimes than the infants demonstrating coordinated feeding at the time of discharge. Continued difficulty with textures at 12 months were also found, along with limited enjoyment of mealtimes, further complicating infant growth, development, and family relationships.[12] In a study of 2118 Taiwanese infants born with a birth weight of less than 2.5 kg who were evaluated in the first 5 years of life, more than 90% of the children were identified with some form of feeding problem in each of the years 2005 and 2006.[13] Of a healthy sample of extremely low birth weight (ELBW) infants examined by Mathisen and colleagues,[14] 80% had feeding problems such as poor intake, fatigue, and delayed feeding skills at 6 months corrected age. These infants were more demanding, more easily frustrated, and more likely to have difficulty with textured foods than the full-term controls.[14] Furthermore, 40% had episodes of aspiration with eating, and 85% continued to have gastroesophageal reflux.[14] Cerro and colleagues[15] studied infants born at less than 32 weeks gestational age, with a mean birth weight of 1243 g, at a mean age of 2.5 years of age (range 1.6–3.6 years). At the time of follow-up they found that 78% of parents were concerned about the quality of food their children were eating, and 45% wished to change their child's eating behaviors.[15] Food refusal was reported by 58% of parents, 51% used food rewards, and 69% used coaxing to encourage intake.[15] In addition, parents reported that 28% had poor weight gain, 33% vomited, 32% were treated with reflux medication, 27% had chronic diarrhea, and 67% constantly refused food.[15]

The risk of poor feeding outcomes appears to increase as gestational age decreases.[14,15] Of ELBW infants weighing 600 g or less, 62% had continued eating problems at 2 years corrected age, and 29% had gastrostomy tubes.[16] These findings justify Thoyre's[17] conclusions that extremely preterm infants may eat sufficiently for discharge but are not yet skilled eaters, and may continue to have major challenges with eating for months and years after discharge from the NICU.

Late preterm (LPT) infants do not escape feeding issues, even though their development is further along than their earlier-born counterparts. Infants born LPT look deceptively vigorous at feeding times, but easily lose state organization and energy to finish eating. These infants typically are less able to achieve effective sucking and swallowing, and may need multiple feeding methods during the transition to oral feeding.[18,19] Breastfeeding is particularly challenging, as these infants are sleepier and have less stamina to latch on and to finish eating. Challenges for feeding are dominant reasons for delayed discharge.[20]

Parents often evaluate their baby's health and their own competency as parents before and after discharge by feeding success and weight gain. Much of an infant's time awake is spent eating in the first year of life. Thoyre[4] found that parents' concerns regarding feeding their infants centered around ensuring adequate intake of volume and calories, safety during feeding, and making changes to the feeding plan once they were home with their infant. Parents report not enjoying the feeding experience,[12] and feeling less confident in caregiving in general and feeding in particular.[21,22] Parents also report having to deal with their infant's variable interest in eating, fatigue, and low intake.[3,4,17,23,24] Feeding disorders in infancy significantly affect the mother-infant interaction,[23] with a higher degree of dysfunction especially when feeding disorders do not have an obvious organic reason. Early feeding disorders contribute more significantly than other regulatory problems to long-term mental health and behavior problems, establishing difficult interaction patterns between parents and children.[25–27] Ongoing infant feeding issues also affect the relationship between the parents themselves.

EATING AS A NEURODEVELOPMENTAL PROCESS

Early infant eating behavior of the infant is thought to be neurologically based and developmental in nature. Several scientists who study the maturational sequence of eating (suck rhythm stability, aggregation of sucks and swallows into runs, length of suck run, and suck-suck interval) suggest that assessment of early eating competence and coordination could predict longer-term neurodevelopmental outcomes,[28–30] and that the coordination of breathing and eating could reflect an "intrinsic calendar of neurodevelopment rather than experiential or learned behavior."[29]

For the purposes of the following discussion, eating refers to the infant's role and feeding refers to the actions taken by the person who provides support for the baby to eat/drink. To eat effectively, infants must sense and react to a variety of tactile, kinesthetic and proprioceptive, olfactory, auditory, and visual inputs at the same time they have to coordinate sucking, swallowing, and breathing. Preterm infants must manage the amount, duration, and timing of sensory input that a feeding demands. In addition, they must maintain an alert state, maintain energy for the duration of feeding, and maintain body as well as oral-motor tone to achieve successful eating. Most early-born infants are not initially able to simultaneously manage these neurodevelopmental demands such that they accomplish successful eating.

DEVELOPMENTAL PRECURSORS FOR SUCCESSFUL EATING

As described in Lickliter elsewhere in this issue, sensory systems develop in an orderly manner, emerging through gestation. Inappropriate inputs at a given developmental stage may interfere with other emerging sensory development.[31] Precursors to infant eating are present early in fetal development. As early as 7 to 8 weeks' gestation there is avoidance in response to perioral stimulation, and by 11 weeks perioral stimulation results in global movement and swallowing. By 16 weeks mouthing can be detected,[31] and by 24 to 25 weeks reflexes such as sucking and rooting can be elicited. By 28 weeks, the fetus can produce a weak suck and palmar grasp,[32] yet stable nonnutritive sucking is not well identified until 34 weeks.[33] Chemosensory development emerges early in gestation, with responsiveness to taste in the amniotic fluid detected by 16 weeks. From 28 to 29 weeks the fetus/newborn can detect, discriminate, and learn about taste and odor (see the articles by Mennella Sullivan elsewhere in this issue, and the reviews by Graven and Browne[34,35]). Newborns orient first to lactating mothers, but quickly begin to differentiate their own mother's breast milk from other breast milk odor.[36,37] Schaal and colleagues[38] examined behavioral responsivity in preterm infants, finding selective response to a mother's familiar odor with orienting to the familiar mother's odor. These contributions to the attachment relationship and to eating success are well documented (see review by Browne and Graven[34] and the article by Sullivan elsewhere in this issue). It is not until the infant is 34 to 36 weeks that safe oral feeding is recommended,[39] and sucking, swallowing, and breathing coordination is not well established until 37 weeks or later.[40]

Successful eating requires coordination of breathing with sucking and swallowing, and involves functional interaction of jaw, tongue, soft palate, pharynx, larynx, and esophagus.[41] Although term infants have appropriate rhythmicity of sucking and swallowing at birth, they continue to show improvement of efficiency over the first month post term age with increased volume per suck.[42,43]

Emerging physiologic studies of eating in preterm infants show a developmental progression with oral-motor skill development between 30 and 45 weeks postmenstrual age. These skills require suction and compression, and the ability to move fluid back into the pharyngeal area and into the esophagus for swallowing. Preceding this skill is nonnutritive sucking (eg, on a finger or a pacifier), which is typically 2 sucks per second, whereas a nutritive suck rhythm and coordination is 1 suck per second. As demonstrated by Mizuno and Ueda,[44] 24 preterm infants studied at 32 weeks postconceptional age had poor sucking pressures, frequencies, duration, and efficiency, with maturation weekly through 36 weeks postconceptional age of all variables. Several other studies similarly have identified a developmental progression of transfer of increasing volumes of milk, rate of transfer, and number of successful oral feedings in preterm infants as they mature to term and postterm ages.[42,45] Gewolb and colleagues[29] found that suck runs in preterm infants were a function of postmenstrual age, not postnatal age, adding to the perspective that success in eating is a neurodevelopmental process. Lau and colleagues[42] demonstrated that preterm infants began nutritive sucking using a weak compression of the nipple, followed by the emergence of negative suction, with a gradual integration and strengthening of both compression and suction noted between 32 and 36 weeks gestational age.

Ultrasound studies show some variability, but most infants mature to a typical ratio of one suck, one swallow, one breath after reaching 37 weeks postconceptional age.[40] The relationship between sucking, swallowing, and breathing matures with increasing postconceptional age.[28,33,44] Infant ventilation stops during swallowing,[46–49] and Durand and colleagues[47] postulate that eating may override respiratory chemical control, further complicating feeding success for infants with respiratory compromise. Hanlon and colleagues[50] examined the effects of feeding on ventilation, and found frequent deglutition apneas with preterm infant feeding and fewer apneas as infants reached term. However, in the infants studied, deglutition apnea was still detected during feeding at term age. Gewolb and Vice[28] further examined respiratory rhythm, integration of swallows, respiratory rhythms, and apneic swallows with feeding preterm infants, finding significant relationships of each with postmenstrual age and not postnatal age.

Taken together, these data indicate that the integration of sucking, swallowing, and breathing is significantly delayed in most infants born preterm compared with infants born at term, that eating skills mature depending on postmenstrual rather than postnatal age regardless of exposure to eating experiences in the preterm infant, that swallows resulting in apnea are typical in early-born infants during eating episodes (potentially setting up a negative reaction to being fed), and that preterm infants may not be able to manage coordinated eating until well after term, especially if they have medical compromise.

In addition to these physiologic aspects of eating, the infant is expected to manage the organization of arousal, which is not well developed until well after term. Motor tone and smooth movements are also not well organized in the preterm infant. Physiologic, state, and motor reactivity to typical sensory input, handling, and social bids can further compromise the infant's availability, vigor, and organization of developing skills for eating and being fed. Repeated negative experiences during eating may lead to feeding aversions, as neuronal mapping is occurring rapidly at this age.[51]

A NEURODEVELOPMENTAL APPROACH TO SUPPORTING EMERGING EATING SKILLS IN HIGH-RISK INFANTS

Adverse short-term and long-term outcomes may be in part attributable to not only a failure of the infant to organize him or herself for successful eating but also to being pushed to eat earlier than they may be able to manage given their level of developmental organization. The emerging understanding of the development of eating skills in high-risk preterm infants and clinical observations of feeding practices in NICUs prompted the development of an approach based on the baby's ability to regulate his or her physiology, level of arousal, motor movements, and management of sensory input as they develop eating skills. Based on the Synactive Theory as an overarching paradigm,[52] the Baby Regulated Organization of Subsystems and Sucking (BROSS) approach encompasses observation of the infant's emerging stability or instability, his or her sensitivity to the physical and handling environment, and determination of the infant's ability to manage skills at 6 consecutive developmental levels of eating. Starting on the first day of admission to the NICU, observation of the infant's organization and vulnerabilities during feeding opportunities is performed, with suggestions for how to support early behavioral organization precursors of emerging pre-eating and eating skills.

At each developmental level of the approach the infant's physiologic, motor, and state systems, or so-called subsystems referred to in the Synactive Theory, are evaluated. Without optimal physiologic organization, appropriate arousal, and robust tone and movement, the infant will not be able to manage appropriate and organized eating skills. During the first phase of the hospitalization, infants born VLBW or ELBW or who are very ill and who are not yet being fed are evaluated for overall stability in these subsystems, and suggestions are made to enhance subsystem organization as described in the Newborn Individualized Developmental Care and Assessment Program (NIDCAP) approach.[53] Positioning, comfort, cyclicity of caregiving, and availability of the familiar mother's sensory offerings is essential at each stage, but in particular when the baby is critically ill and typically disorganized. The first stage of the BROSS is thus described as Subsystems Stability in Bed, during typical NICU interactions and procedures.

As the baby becomes more stable and is able to be handled and perhaps held by his or her parents or professional staff, the same evaluation is made of Stability of Subsystems when Handled. This stage typically occurs when the infant has developed some medical stability but is still not robust enough for any introduction of oral feedings. Transfer from the bed to the lap, holding by a sensitive caregiver, and provision of feeding-related cues such as smells of milk, elicitation of the rooting reflex, and sound of the caregiver's voice can assist the infant in foundational readiness for eating. Holding during all feedings once stability is achieved, even if the infant receives gavage feedings, supports the infant as he or she develops an expectation of organized external sensory input from the caregiver, and assists with organization of the infant's competence during feeding. Often infants who can manage to have some stability while held are unable to manage multiple sensory inputs at the same time, much less being prompted to suck either nutritively or nonnutritively. Mosca[54] demonstrated that holding stable premature infants during gavage feedings helped the infant to increase the time they spent in more desirable, quiet alert, and drowsy infant behavioral states, resulted in less apnea at the beginning of feedings than seen when infants were fed prone in bed, and did not compromise infant physiologic stability. Behavioral states become significantly more organized across the 31-week to term gestational ages.[55]

Once the infant is predictably able to show subsystem stability while held and shows more robust and consistent indications of hunger through the rooting reflex, mouthing, increased activity, and responsiveness to the mothers voice and odor, they are able to progress to Stability of Subsystems During Nonnutritive Sucking on a finger, pacifier, or a mother's empty breast as the next developmental phase. As the infant matures, nonnutritive sucking (NNS) becomes more robust and stable, optimally organizing at around 34 weeks.[33] When first introduced, NNS may be weak or disorganized, with the infant rarely able to keep the pacifier in his or her mouth. As the baby's subsystems become more stable and they can organize their arousal, breathing, and motor tone, a stronger and more rhythmic sucking pattern will emerge with 5 to 10 or more sucks per burst. During NNS there is no need for the baby to swallow, making it easier to breathe while sucking.

Infants may become very predictable and robust in their NNS patterns and may use NNS for calming. However, robustness of NNS is not predictive of infants' ability to transition to managing fluid,[56] as they then must protect their airway and coordinate sucking, swallowing, and breathing. Many infants approach a nutritive bottle with an NNS pattern, but when the fluid is introduced into their posterior pharynx they exhibit deglutition apnea, as described previously. This Obligatory phase can be very challenging for the infant, as it is a significant developmental transition in the progression to oral feeding. It can be particularly challenging if the person feeding the infant is not in tune with the infant's sucking, and lack of breathing and can result in severe physiologic compromise. Many infants suck in 10- to 20-suck bursts without breathing, as if they were sucking nonnutritively without the need to coordinate swallowing and breathing. Once the infant starts to breathe he or she often cannot manage the fluid that has been expressed during the sucking burst. Attunement of the feeder to the subsystem organization is essential in helping the infant avoid decompensation and, importantly, avoid a negative experience with eating. Often infants need a slowed flow from the nipple, frequent rest periods, and significant pacing to manage even minimal amounts of fluid, all of which have been shown to be beneficial when an infant is struggling to manage the suck-swallow-breathe coordination.[57–59] However, many infants who exhibit extreme physiologic, state, or motor compromise consistent with this phase should not be orally fed, but should instead be allowed to mature for several days to weeks at the NNS phase to allow for development of skills.

As infants mature, they develop an increasingly adaptive response to managing the flow of fluid from the nipple, and show an Alternating Pattern of sucking and breathing. That is, they suck for a burst of 3 to 5 sucks and alternate with breathing, albeit tachypneically. In this phase, initially there frequently are longer sucking bursts accompanied by mild desaturations, with recovery during the tachypneic catch up. Later in this phase the sucking bursts and tachypneic catch-up breaths are shorter in duration as the infant begins to better manage the suck, swallow, and breathe coordination. Typical of this phase is limited state availability and motor robustness to complete the amount expected to be fed.

The Intermittent Sucking Phase indicates further developmental organization and management of subsystems during eating. The infant inserts brief catch breaths once every 2 to 3 sucks, and longer sucking bursts appear with the catch breaths imbedded. Suction on the nipple becomes stronger, and there is an integration of suction and expression. Ultimately, there is a longer burst and more efficient sucking, with greater volumes of fluid transferred to be swallowed. The infant begins to have a more robust alert state for eating, and may be available for some mild social interaction.

The hallmark of the Coordinated Phase is when the infant develops a mature and coordinated sucking pattern with sucking bursts of 20 to 30 sucks, seamlessly integrating breathing with sucking and swallowing. Although many infants have a pattern of one suck, one swallow, and one breath, most babies develop their own coordinated pattern with modulated suction and expression. The alert state becomes more robust for the entire feeding, and more predictable availability for social interaction begins to emerge. This phase is typically seen in infants after transitioning home from the NICU.

Further eating organization, smoothness, and predictability of eating routines and social relationship development occurs well after term for most infants. The Integrated Phase is described as having full coordination of sucking/swallowing and breathing without increased work of breathing or tachypnea, clear demands to be fed and enjoyment of eating, and unique social interaction characteristics between the baby and the primary caregiver.

Pilot data collected for 30 preterm infants (not adjusted for medical morbidity) in a cross-sectional pilot study reveals a correlation between increasing postmenstrual age and increasing feeding score (Spearman's correlation yielded a rho of 0.68 [$P<.0001$]).[60] This correlation suggests that an increasingly organized feeding score is correlated with increasing postmenstrual age at the time of the observation.

CHALLENGES TO EMERGING EATING COMPETENCE FOR HIGH-RISK INFANTS

The described phases of the development of eating skills are typically observed in preterm infants who have medical histories with few complications. However, no ranges of gestational ages are offered because of the unique individual developmental course that each infant experiences. In general, the descriptors follow the findings of physiologic and behavioral developmental studies. Although most infants follow this general pattern of development of eating skills, many infants have a slower progress than others and may take days, weeks, or months until they achieve the same level of eating that other infants born at the same conceptional age achieve. Contributions to these delays may include the medical condition of the infant, including early birth, invasive and noninvasive interventions in the NICU that may disturb the organization of the already compromised infant, and the environment in which the infant is developing. Infants with more medical comorbidities are most at risk for delayed attainment of oral feedings.[61] Dodrill and colleagues[62] studied 472 infants born at less than 37 weeks gestational age, and found that preterm infants who were less mature at birth, or who had a greater number of medical comorbidities, were delayed in their transition to full oral feedings and were more mature at attainment of full oral feedings. The earlier born or medically fragile the infant and the longer he or she is exposed to these 3 factors, the more likely it is that eating organization will be affected. For example, studies on outcomes of chronically ill and hospitalized groups of children show several similar findings; that the smaller the infant was at birth and the longer he or she was ventilated or had major surgery, the less weight they gained after discharge.[7] For infants with bronchopulmonary dysplasia, successful full oral feedings typically not only delayed but are negatively correlated with the gestational age of the infant, with later development occurring for those infants born more prematurely.[61] Similarly, infants with cardiac defects had significant delays with feeding readiness, successful gastric feeding, oromotor readiness, and oromotor skills.[61,63]

Effects of the infant medical condition on successful eating outcomes include pain and discomfort that is internally generated, such as abdominal pain or headaches, which are difficult to understand in the preverbal infant; nausea or gastrointestinal upset such as gastroesophageal reflux; respiratory distress and what adults would describe as breathlessness; pharmacologic side effects; neurochemical imbalance; and nutritional deficits, among others. The extent to which infants associate discomfort and pain with being fed is not known. However, what is known is that infants with gastrointestinal issues as well as those with respiratory disease are overrepresented in tertiary feeding clinics.[64–66]

Procedures can also affect the infant's success at eating. Infants typically undergo unpredictable interventions, which often override the infant's physiologic stability; timing of procedures that either interrupt or do not take into consideration the infant's sleep state; pain and discomfort from procedures with limited or no pain management; lack of basic comfort measures such as positioning for self-regulation; and prolonged intubation and feeding tubes. Prolonged use of nasogastric tubes, for instance, is correlated with increased episodes of gastroesophageal reflux, as well as feeding problems and increased facial defensive behaviors in infants well after discharge from the NICU.[67,68]

Accumulating evidence of the impact of environments on infant organization primarily highlights the lack of the regulating environment of the mother's body, so important for most infants during feeding interactions (see the articles by Mennella, Sullivan, and Champagne elsewhere in this issue). Furthermore it has long been known that environments filled with unpredictable and intrusive sound, light, and activity can affect the infant's physiologic and state organization.[69] Other factors that influence the infant's organization for eating are nonsupportive bedding and handling that do not allow for self-regulation and deep sleep, and multiple caregivers who present a variety of unfamiliar odors, voices, touch, and rhythm to which the infant must adjust.

RECOMMENDATIONS FOR FEEDING HIGH-RISK INFANTS IN THE NICU AND BEYOND

Although many challenges to successful feeding of premature and high-risk newborns have been identified, and more information is available about the neurodevelopmental processes that contribute to eating success, there still is no consistent approach to intervention strategies that may ameliorate the short-term and long-term adverse outcomes of feeding high-risk infants.[7,55] However, the developmental sequence of infant organization for eating is now being recognized, and an informed approach to supporting development of infant organization in all areas of development seems prudent. Support for early and individualized organization of physiology, state, and motor tone and movement, the substrates of all developmental skills is necessary both in the NICU and while the infant and family are followed at home.

In the NICU, protection from an intrusive environment, provision of a familiar and consistent caregiver (in most instances the parents), provision of uninterrupted rest periods, attention to the infant when he or she is available behaviorally, protection from unwarranted and disorganizing procedures, and attention to organizing procedures such as holding while eating are foundations for successful eating. Recognition of the developmental nature of acquisition of eating skills, and not pushing the infant further than he or she is developmentally capable of at any given time, is essential. To accomplish this sensitivity, a thorough knowledge of infant behavioral communication of his or her capabilities and challenges is necessary, along with a willingness to modify the expectations of successful eating from the amount the baby is fed to the quality of the feeding.

Finally, and likely most importantly, supporting the parent-infant relationship and assisting the parents to feel competent with the feeding their baby is of utmost importance. As detailed earlier, much of the development of eating skills is accomplished after discharge from the NICU. Coupled with the significant incidence of both short-term and long-term growth and feeding failures in high-risk infants, more attention needs to be given to the development of eating and feeding competence of the parent-infant dyad, both in the NICU and as they transition to their family home.

SUMMARY

The short-term and long-term adverse growth and eating behavior outcomes of early-born and high-risk babies reveal major challenges for professionals, infants, and parents in both the NICU and community settings. Research indicates that eating is a complex and ongoing physiologic and behavioral achievement for growing neonates, and that recognition of this neurodevelopmental process can inform current feeding practices. A clinically informed approach to recognition of infant behavioral organization by development of the subsystems of physiologic, arousal, and motor areas is presented as a means by which professionals and parents can assist the infant's ability to have more organized eating experiences. Finally, recommendations for practices that recognize the neurodevelopmental processes and the need for competent, relationship-based eating opportunities between parents and infants are proposed.

REFERENCES

1. Hospital discharge of the high-risk neonate—proposed guidelines. American Academy of Pediatrics. Committee on Fetus and Newborn. Pediatrics 1998; 102(2 Pt 1):411–7.

2. Silberstein D, Geva R, Feldman R, et al. The transition to oral feeding in low-risk premature infants: relation to infant neurobehavioral functioning and mother-infant feeding interaction. Early Hum Dev 2009;85(3):157–62.

3. Pridham K, Saxe R, Limbo R. Feeding issues for mothers of very low-birth-weight premature infants through the first year. J Perinat Neonatal Nurs 2004;18(2):161–9.

4. Thoyre SM. Challenges mothers identify in bottle feeding their preterm infants. Neonatal Netw 2001;20(1):41–50.

5. Wood NS, Costeloe K, Gibson AT, et al. The EPICure study: growth and associated problems in children born at 25 weeks of gestational age or less. Arch Dis Child Fetal Neonatal Ed 2003;88(6):F492–500.

6. Ehrenkranz RA, Dusick AM, Vohr BR, et al. Growth in the neonatal intensive care unit influences neurodevelopmental and growth outcomes of extremely low birth weight infants. Pediatrics 2006;117(4):1253–61.

7. Ross ES, Krebs N, Shroyer AL, et al. Early growth faltering in healthy term infants predicts longitudinal growth. Early Hum Dev 2009;85:583–8.

8. Deloian B. Caring connections: Nursing support transitioning premature infants and their families home from the hospital. Denver (CO): University of Colorado Health Sciences Center, School of Nursing; 1998.

9. Ross E. Ensuring feeding success after NICU discharge: eating well enough versus eating well. Developmental interventions in neonatal care. Washington, DC, November 7, 2009.

10. Dusick AM, Poindexter BB, Ehrenkranz RA, et al. Growth failure in the preterm infant: can we catch up? Semin Perinatol 2003;27(4):302–10.

11. Dodrill P, Cleghorn G, Donovan T, et al. Growth patterns in preterm infants born appropriate for gestational age. J Paediatr Child Health 2008;44(6):332–7.

12. Hawdon JM, Beauregard N, Slattery J, et al. Identification of neonates at risk of developing feeding problems in infancy. Dev Med Child Neurol 2000;42(4): 235–9.

13. Howe TH, Hsu CH, Tsai MW. Prevalence of feeding related issues/difficulties in Taiwanese children with history of prematurity, 2003-2006. Res Dev Disabil 2010;31(2):510–6.

14. Mathisen B, Worrall L, O'Callaghan M, et al. Feeding problems and dysphagia in six-month-old extremely low birth weight infants. Adv Speech Lang Pathol 2000; 2(1):9–17.

15. Cerro N, Zeunert S, Simmer KN, et al. Eating behaviour of children 1.5-3.5 years born preterm: parents' perceptions. J Paediatr Child Health 2002;38(1):72–8.

16. Sweet MP, Hodgman JE, Pena I, et al. Two-year outcome of infants weighing 600 grams or less at birth and born 1994 through 1998. Obstet Gynecol 2003;101(1): 18–23.

17. Thoyre S. Feeding outcomes of extremely premature infants after neonatal care. J Obstet Gynecol Neonatal Nurs 2007;36(4):366–76.

18. Bakewell-Sachs S. Near-term/late preterm infants. Newborn Infant Nurs Rev 2007;7(2):67–71.

19. Engle WA, Tomashek KM, Wallman C. "Late-preterm" infants: a population at risk. Pediatrics 2007;120(6):1390–401.

20. Kirkby S, Greenspan JS, Kornhauser M, et al. Clinical outcomes and cost of the moderately preterm infant. Adv Neonatal Care 2007;7(2):80–7.

21. Docherty SL, Miles MS, Holditch-Davis D. Worry about child health in mothers of hospitalized medically fragile infants. Adv Neonatal Care 2002;2(2):84–92.

22. Miles MS, Holditch-Davis D, Burchinal P, et al. Distress and growth outcomes in mothers of medically fragile infants. Nurs Res 1999;48(3):129–40.

23. Lucarelli L, Ambruzzi AM, Cimino S, et al. Feeding disorders in infancy: an empirical study on mother-infant interactions. Minerva Pediatr 2003;55(3):243–53, 253–9.

24. Kavanaugh K, Mead L, Meier P, et al. Getting enough: mother's concerns about breastfeeding a premature infant after discharge. J Obstet Gynecol Neonatal Nurs 1995;24(1):23–32.

25. Hagekull B, Dahl M. Infants with and without feeding difficulties: maternal experiences. Int J Eat Disord 1987;6(1):83–98.

26. Schmid G, Schreier A, Meyer R, et al. A prospective study on the persistence of infant crying, sleeping and feeding problems and preschool behaviour. Acta Paediatr 2010;99(2):286–90.

27. Hagekull B, Bohlin G, Rydell AM. Maternal sensitivity, infant temperament, and the development of early feeding problems. Infant Ment Health J 1997;18(1):92–106.

28. Gewolb IH, Vice FL. Maturational changes in the rhythms, patterning, and coordination of respiration and swallow during feeding in preterm and term infants. Dev Med Child Neurol 2006;48(7):589–94.

29. Gewolb IH, Vice FL, Schwietzer-Kenney EL, et al. Developmental patterns of rhythmic suck and swallow in preterm infants. Dev Med Child Neurol 2001; 43(1):22–7.

30. Medoff-Cooper B, Shults J, Kaplan J. Sucking behavior of preterm neonates as a predictor of developmental outcomes. J Dev Behav Pediatr 2009;30(1):16–22.

31. Miller JL, Sonies BC, Macedonia C. Emergence of oropharyngeal, laryngeal and swallowing activity in the developing fetal upper aerodigestive tract: an ultrasound evaluation. Early Hum Dev 2003;71(1):61–87.

32. Lecanuet JP, Jacquet AY. Fetal responsiveness to maternal passive swinging in low heart rate variability state: effects of stimulation direction and duration. Dev Psychobiol 2002;40(1):57–67.

33. Hack M, Estabrook MM, Robertson SS. Development of sucking rhythm in preterm infants. Early Hum Dev 1985;11(2):133–40.

34. Graven S, Browne J. Sensory development in the fetus, neonate, and infant: introduction and overview. Newborn Infant Nurs Rev 2008;8(4):169–72.

35. Browne J. Chemosensory development of the fetus and newborn. Newborn Infant Nurs Rev 2008;8(4):180–6.

36. Porter RH, Winberg J. Unique salience of maternal breast odors for newborn infants. Neurosci Biobehav Rev 1999;23(3):439–49.

37. Winberg J, Porter RH. Olfaction and human neonatal behaviour: clinical implications. Acta Paediatr 1998;87(1):6–10.

38. Schaal B, Hummel T, Soussignan R. Olfaction in the fetal and premature infant: functional status and clinical implications. Clin Perinatol 2004;31(2):261–85, vi–vii.

39. Simpson C, Schanler RJ, Lau C. Early introduction of oral feeding in preterm infants. Pediatrics 2002;110(3):517–22.

40. Bu'Lock F, Woolridge MW, Baum JD. Development of co-ordination of sucking, swallowing and breathing: ultrasound study of term and preterm infants. Dev Med Child Neurol 1990;32(8):669–78.

41. Wolf L, Glass R. Feeding and swallowing disorders in infancy. Tucson (AZ): Therapy Skill Builders; 1992.

42. Lau C, Alagugurusamy R, Schanler RJ, et al. Characterization of the developmental stages of sucking in preterm infants during bottle feeding. Acta Paediatr 2000;89(7):846–52.

43. Qureshi MA, Vice FL, Taciak VL, et al. Changes in rhythmic suckle feeding patterns in term infants in the first month of life. Dev Med Child Neurol 2002; 44(1):34–9.

44. Mizuno K, Ueda A. The maturation and coordination of sucking, swallowing, and respiration in preterm infants. J Pediatr 2003;142(1):36–40.

45. Medoff-Cooper B, Ratcliffe SJ. Development of preterm infants: feeding behaviors and Brazelton neonatal behavioral assessment scale at 40 and 44 weeks' postconceptional age. ANS Adv Nurs Sci 2005;28(4):356–63.

46. al-Sayed LE, Schrank WI, Thach BT. Ventilatory sparing strategies and swallowing pattern during bottle feeding in human infants. J Appl Physiol 1994;77(1):78–83.

47. Durand M, Leahy FN, MacCallum M, et al. Effect of feeding on the chemical control of breathing in the newborn infant. Pediatr Res 1981;15(12):1509–12.

48. Selley WG, Ellis RE, Flack FC, et al. Coordination of sucking, swallowing and breathing in the newborn: its relationship to infant feeding and normal development. Br J Disord Commun 1990;25(3):311–27.

49. Tarrant SC, Ellis RE, Flack FC, et al. Comparative review of techniques for recording respiratory events at rest and during deglutition. Dysphagia 1997;12(1):24–38.

50. Hanlon MB, Tripp JH, Ellis RE, et al. Deglutition apnoea as indicator of maturation of suckle feeding in bottle-fed preterm infants. Dev Med Child Neurol 1997;39(8):534–42.

51. Edelman GM. Neural Darwinism. The theory of neuronal group selection. New York: Basic Books, Inc; 1987.

52. Als H. Toward a synactive theory of development: promise for the assessment and support of infant individuality. Infant Ment Health J 1982;3(4):229–43.

53. Als H, Gibes R. Newborn individualized developmental care and assessment program (NIDCAP). Training guide. Boston: Children's Hospital; 1990.

54. Mosca N. Holding premature infants during gavage feeding: effect on apnea, bradycardia, oxygenation, gastric residual, gastrin, and behavioral state. Cleveland (OH): Case Western Reserve University; 1995.

55. Foreman SW, Thomas KA, Blackburn ST. Individual and gender differences matter in preterm infant state development. J Obstet Gynecol Neonatal Nurs 2008;37(6):657–65.

56. Mizuno K, Ueda A. Development of sucking behavior in infants who have not been fed for 2 months after birth. Pediatr Int 2001;43(3):251–5.

57. Chang YJ, Lin CP, Lin YJ, et al. Effects of single-hole and cross-cut nipple units on feeding efficiency and physiological parameters in premature infants. J Nurs Res 2007;15(3):215–23.

58. Lau C, Schanler RJ. Oral feeding in premature infants: advantage of a self-paced milk flow. Acta Paediatr 2000;89(4):453–9.

59. Law-Morstatt L, Judd DM, Snyder P, et al. Pacing as a treatment technique for transitional sucking patterns. J Perinatol 2003;23(6):483–8.

60. Ross E, Browne J. Baby Regulated Organization of Systems and Sucking (BROSS). The physical and developmental environment of the high-risk infant. Clearwater, FL, January 28, 2002.

61. Jadcherla SR, Wang M, Vijayapal AS, et al. Impact of prematurity and co-morbidities on feeding milestones in neonates: a retrospective study. J Perinatol 2010;30(3):201–8.

62. Dodrill P, Donovan T, Cleghorn G, et al. Attainment of early feeding milestones in preterm neonates. J Perinatol 2008;28(8):549–55.

63. Medoff-Cooper B, Naim M, Torowicz D, et al. Feeding, growth, and nutrition in children with congenitally malformed hearts. Cardiol Young 2010;20(Suppl 3):149–53.

64. Burklow KA, McGrath AM, Valerius KS, et al. Relationship between feeding difficulties, medical complexity, and gestational age. Nutr Clin Pract 2002;17(6): 373–8.

65. Field D, Garland M, Williams K. Correlates of specific childhood feeding problems. J Paediatr Child Health 2003;39(4):299–304.

66. Rommel N, De Meyer AM, Feenstra L, et al. The complexity of feeding problems in 700 infants and young children presenting to a tertiary care institution. J Pediatr Gastroenterol Nutr 2003;37(1):75–84.

67. Dodrill P, McMahon S, Ward E, et al. Long-term oral sensitivity and feeding skills of low-risk pre-term infants. Early Hum Dev 2004;76(1):23–37.

68. Peter CS, Wiechers C, Bohnhorst B, et al. Influence of nasogastric tubes on gastroesophageal reflux in preterm infants: a multiple intraluminal impedance study. J Pediatr 2002;141(2):277–9.

69. Long JG, Philip AG, Lucey JF. Excessive handling as a cause of hypoxemia. Pediatrics 1980;65(2):203–7.

Designing Environments for Developmental Care

Robert D. White, MD

KEYWORDS

- NICU design • Developmental care • Family-centered care
- Skin-to-skin care • Single-family room

The environment of care has been recognized as an important factor in the healing process for centuries. This is true for all individuals but none more so than newborn infants, for whom the hospital is not only a place of healing but also where an extraordinary and unique period of growth and development must occur—it cannot wait until after the infant is well and discharged home.

An attempt to define the optimal environment of care is not as simple as replicating the in utero environment. The infant is no longer in utero, and therefore some physiologic and developmental needs have changed, for example, the circadian signals experienced by the fetus, which include transplacental hormones as well as maternal body temperature and activity, have been removed. Second, even if it were desirable, replication of the in utero environment is not entirely possible, for example, suspension of the infant in an enclosed, fluid-filled container, with all nutrients being delivered via the umbilical vein and toxins removed via the umbilical artery is beyond our current capabilities.

We are forced, then, to suggest the optimal environment for infant development in the hospital setting from 3 bodies of knowledge: (1) direct evidence from hospital-based studies, (2) extrapolation from what the environment is in utero, and (3) from extensive animal studies, knowing that animal developmental stages are always a bit different than those of the human infant. What seems certain, in general terms, is that extended intimate contact with the mother, facilitation of sleep, and protection from toxins are important. In most other areas, we have to make our best educated guess, because, for better or worse, preterm infants are being exposed to the environment that we design for them—we cannot suspend decision making until better data are presented. The status quo for most neonatal intensive care units (NICUs) was not based on any developmental data, but on technological and financial imperatives, so any consideration in this regard is likely to be an improvement.

Financial disclosure/conflicts of interest: The author has nothing to disclose.
Regional Newborn Program, Pediatrix Medical Group, Memorial Hospital, 615 North Michigan Street, South Bend, IN 46601, USA
E-mail address: Robert_White@pediatrix.com

Clin Perinatol 38 (2011) 745–749
doi:10.1016/j.clp.2011.08.012   **perinatology.theclinics.com**
0095-5108/11/$ – see front matter © 2011 Elsevier Inc. All rights reserved.

OPTIMAL ENVIRONMENTAL DESIGN, BASED ON CURRENT KNOWLEDGE
General Considerations

There is solid reason to believe that the best environment for neurodevelopment of the newborn is provided by intimate and extended contact with the mother, often referred to as kangaroo or skin-to-skin (STS) care, which closely resembles the in utero stimuli that are biologically anticipated by the fetal brain. Even STS care with someone other than the mother or being held fully clothed provides a "living" environment that is far more developmentally appropriate than the inert, artificial environment provided by an incubator or warmer.[1]

Clinical evidence that STS care improves outcomes in high-risk infants has only recently been reported,[2] although studies in animals, referred to in some detail in other articles in this issue, establish that prolonged and intimate contact of a baby with its mother is vital.

Design of the NICU to enhance the likelihood of STS care involves, most importantly, sufficient space and furnishings so that parents can stay and interact with their baby for extended periods of time in comfort. In most Western cultures, this also includes provision for some degree of visual and auditory privacy. The primary design strategy that allows extended periods of contact between a baby and his or her parents is the single-family room (SFR), so-called because it emphasizes the importance of the family unit, especially when that involves twins or higher-order multiple births. It is clear that the SFR is preferred by most parents and caregivers,[3–7] and evidence is now accumulating that it also leads to better outcomes for babies.[2,8] Developmentally, the SFR design not only facilitates provision of the optimal developmental microenvironment for the infant STS, but also increases the likelihood that elements of the macroenvironment, such as noise and light, can be better controlled.

Protection of the newborn infant from toxins includes those that emanate from the built environment, those that are used transiently during care or general contact, and infectious agents. Many potential substances can be present in the hospital environment, such as volatile organic compounds[9] and electromagnetic radiation.[10] Additional substances may be introduced via the airborne (eg, alcohol wipes, cleaning fluid vapors, particulate dust) or contact route (eg, chlorhexidine or iodine-containing solutions for cleansing skin or wounds), or directly placed within the body (eg, plasticizers in feeding tubes and intravenous materials). Infectious agents can also reach the baby in each of these 3 ways. It is apparent that good design entails consideration of these issues, and is relevant to our topic to the extent that the toxins affect the developmental status of the infant directly (as with fragrant or noxious odors) or indirectly (as with effects of any toxin on cellular growth and development in the brain). Building codes, such as the Recommended Standards for Newborn ICU Design,[11] address these concerns in the built environment. Control of toxins that are introduced into the environment is usually straightforward once a substance is identified as a toxin, but substances with an odor or taste that may influence infant behavior and development may not be identified as a toxin, and will be discussed later in this article.

Developmentally appropriate lighting in the NICU requires the ability to adjust to the infant's developmental stage. There is no evidence that visual stimulation is required at any point before term, although it is clear that infants respond to direct light as if it were noxious and to faces as if they were of interest many weeks before term. There is considerable evidence, though, that providing light in a circadian cycle is beneficial to infants (see the article by Dr Gravens, elsewhere in this issue), at least once the neural structures (retinohypothalamic tract, suprachiasmatic nuclei) that carry this information from the eye to the brain are formed. A more detailed review of lighting considerations in the NICU has recently been published.[12]

Avoiding noxious sounds in the NICU while facilitating developmentally beneficial auditory stimuli is a challenge, because much of the therapy we provide is intrinsically noisy. Monitors, respiratory support, movement of equipment, and even the multitude of human voices serve an important purpose and cannot be completely eliminated. Use of the SFR to reduce environmental noise and facilitate exposure to maternal sounds helps to some extent, as does large spaces between babies, because sound transmission declines geometrically as distances are increased. Once these major factors have been addressed, though, further noise control requires specific design features discussed later in this article. When the baby's environment has been made as quiet as possible, there remains considerable uncertainty as to what, if anything, should be introduced to provide developmental benefit to the baby when the parents are not present. Music in particular has been explored, but although there is enough evidence to say that the topic is worth further exploration, there is not enough to say what source, type, intensity, or duration of music is beneficial to preterm infants.

The NICU environment is particularly bereft of developmentally appropriate touch and kinesthetic stimuli unless the baby is being held. Our usual care routines involve a great deal of unpleasant touch and movement for infants, and there is little that can be done with the built environment, short of encouraging parental presence to change this.

The chemosensory (smell, taste) environment in the NICU is also one where there is little that can be done with design features. Perhaps the most important consideration for those who are building units at this time is to be open to the possibility that certain odors may influence caregiver and parental sense of well-being, as has been demonstrated in other settings.

DESIGN FEATURES THAT PROMOTE DEVELOPMENTAL CARE

It is evident from the preceding discussion that proper NICU design must facilitate intimate and extended parental presence. The incubator or warmer will never be more than a meager alternative to this simple, natural, unique environment already well designed for the purpose of nurturing the well or ill infant. It should also be apparent that, at least in most Western cultures, this family environment is best provided in the SFR setting.

Encouraging and facilitating family presence is difficult in any space smaller than 180 square feet. The room must be 10 to 14 feet wide to accommodate patient care with sufficient clearance for movement of equipment and personnel. The patient care space, which would include both a comfortable chair for STS care and the patient bed (incubator, warmer, or bassinette), direct care equipment, supplies that must be at the bedside, and clearance for circulation necessitates a space that is at least 10 feet in the other dimension. Another 4 feet is needed on one side (usually oriented toward the aisle or hallway) for additional storage, waste containers, and a handwashing sink, and at least 4 feet is needed on the other side for family space, although 6 to 8 feet will be much more conducive to comfortable extended stays. Thus, the minimum dimensions for an SFR room should be 10 × 18 feet, and a more desirable room to promote family presence and participation would be at least 12 × 20 feet, and ideally up to 280 square feet. Rooms to accommodate twins would require less than twice this amount, because some supplies and all the family space are already provided; 360 square feet would be suitable for this purpose. Further details about the needs of the patient room can be found elsewhere[11]; for the purpose of this article, the key aspect is that the room must be large enough and properly equipped to encourage and facilitate extended parental interaction with the infant.

Ambient lighting in the patient care space should avoid the possibility that a baby would ever be positioned facing directly into a light source, whether daylight or electric lighting. Direct light is unpleasant to patients of any age who are trying to sleep, so rooms for babies who cannot block light out through their thin eyelids, may not be able to turn away from the light, and cannot communicate their needs must have only indirect ambient lighting.

Establishing a circadian rhythm for ambient lighting can be done with electric lighting alone, or with a combination of electric light and daylight. Although the absolute levels of light, the amount of change in light levels from day to night, and the duration of brighter light needed to entrain the circadian system are not clearly defined for newborns, the studies that showed that circadian changes in lighting had an impact on newborns typically used daylight levels of at least 300 lux for at least 8 hours, with a decrement at night of at least 200 lux from the daytime level.

Sound levels in the patient care area should not exceed 50 dB most of the time to facilitate infant sleep, and to allow the baby to easily hear human voices at normal conversational levels.[13] Simply providing private rooms does not guarantee that this level of quiet can be reached, although it does make it much easier.[14] Even in private rooms, attention to space (largest floor space and highest ceilings possible) and surfaces (acoustical ceiling tile, resilient flooring; sound-absorbing wall surfaces where possible) is important. For infants who are cared for in multibed rooms, the elements of space, sound-reducing and absorbing surfaces, and structures that baffle rather than reflect sound are even more critical.

A great deal of sound can be removed from the NICU by thoughtful design of traffic patterns and workspaces. For example, containers for trash, used linens, and recyclables that are located against the wall and can be accessed through a panel in the hallway will reduce traffic into the patient room; it may also be possible to resupply certain storage areas within the patient room with this strategy as well. Beds that are designed around a perimeter rather than down a long hallway will reduce travel time for staff, and decrease the noise levels for the beds at the near end of the hallway.

Communication devices are now available that markedly reduce audible equipment alarms, cross-unit conversations, and paging/intercom noise. Reduction in equipment noise has been more difficult to achieve, although some manufacturers are paying greater attention to the noise generated by incubators and respiratory devices in particular, so incorporating this element into equipment selection is worthwhile.

NOT FAR INTO THE FUTURE...

Our units, until now built around commercial infant beds and high technology, are likely to be increasingly centered around the concept that active family participation in care is essential to optimizing neonatal outcomes. It is also likely that we will recognize the baby's brain as worthy of even more attention than the lungs, heart, and other organs on which our attention had been focused in the early days of neonatology.

We are on the verge of having several devices that give us a real-time picture of the effects of our interventions and environmental stimuli on the infant brain. Until now, we have had to depend on infant cues and long-term follow-up, and although both are powerful and important tools, they are incomplete. Those who are designing NICUs for the future should anticipate bedside monitors that tell us as much or more about the status of the infant brain as we have come to expect from our current generation of cardiorespiratory monitors. Units themselves, then, should be designed for considerable flexibility—in lighting levels, in noise control and sound enhancements, and, of course, in family participation in care.

The developmentally appropriate NICU of the future will not just prepare the baby for home, it will prepare home for the baby. Caregivers will still need technical expertise, but to a far greater extent will be teaching, encouraging, and facilitating family participation in care. The NICU of this future era will have better technology than our current units, yet it will be in the background—tiny, quiet, and efficient—allowing the "feel" of the unit to be closer to that of a multifamily home than of an ICU. After all, as pointed out at the outset of this article, the current NICU environment was not the result of evidence that the sights, sounds, and feeling we currently experience are beneficial to babies, and we now know the contrary to be true. This change is already well under way, and the outlines of the NICU of 2020 are starting to take shape.

REFERENCES

1. White RD. The newborn intensive care unit environment of care: how we got here, where we're headed, and why. Semin Perinatol 2011;35:2–7.
2. Ortenstrand A, Westrup B, Brostrom EB, et al. The Stockholm neonatal family-centered care study: effects on length of stay and infant morbidity. Pediatrics 2010;125:e278–85.
3. Smith TJ, Schoenbeck K, Clayton S. Staff perceptions of work quality of a neonatal intensive care unit before and after transition from an open bay to a private room design. Work 2009;33:211–27.
4. Cone SK, Short S, Gutcher G. From "Baby Barn" to the "single family room designed NICU": a report of staff perceptions one year post occupancy. Newborn Infant Nurs Rev 2010;10:97–103.
5. Shepley MM, Harris DD, White R. Open-bay and single family room neonatal intensive care units: caregiver satisfaction and stress. Environ Behav 2008;40:249–68.
6. Stevens DC, Helseth CC, Khan MA, et al. Neonatal intensive care nursery staff perceive enhanced workplace quality with the single-family room design. J Perinatol 2010;30:352–8.
7. Carter BS, Carter A, Bennett S. Families' views upon experiencing change in the neonatal intensive care unit environment from the "baby barn" to the private room. J Perinatol 2008;28:827–9.
8. Domanico R, Davis DK, Coleman F, et al. Documenting the NICU design dilemma: comparative patient progress in open-ward and single-family room units. J Perinatol 2011;31:281–8.
9. Marshall-Baker A. Healthful environments for hospitalized infants. HERD 2011;4:127–41.
10. Bellieni CV, Acampa M, Maffei M, et al. Electromagnetic fields produced by incubators influence heart rate variability in newborns. Arch Dis Child Fetal Neonatal Ed 2008;93:F298–301.
11. White RD. Recommended standards for the newborn ICU. J Perinatol 2007;27:S4–19.
12. Rizzo P, Rea M, White R. Lighting for today's neonatal intensive care unit. Newborn Infant Nurs Rev 2010;10:107–13.
13. Philbin MK. Planning the acoustic environment of a neonatal intensive care unit. Clin Perinatol 2004;31:331–52.
14. Stevens DC, Akram Khan M, Munson DP, et al. The impact of architectural design upon the environmental sound and light exposure of neonates who require intensive care: an evaluation of the Boekelheide Neonatal Intensive Care Nursery. J Perinatol 2007;27(Suppl 2):S20–8.

Index

Note: Page numbers of article titles are in **boldface** type.

Clin Perinatol 38 (2011) 751–758
doi:10.1016/S0095-5108(11)00118-7
0095-5108/11/$ – see front matter © 2011 Elsevier Inc. All rights reserved.

perinatology.theclinics.com

United States Postal Service

Statement of Ownership, Management, and Circulation
(All Periodicals Publications Except Requestor Publications)

1. Publication Title	2. Publication Number								3. Filing Date
Clinics in Perinatology	0	0	1	-	7	4	4	4	9/16/11

4. Issue Frequency	5. Number of Issues Published Annually	6. Annual Subscription Price
Mar, Jun, Sep, Dec	4	$256.00

7. Complete Mailing Address of Known Office of Publication (Not printer) (Street, city, county, state, and ZIP+4®)

Elsevier Inc.
360 Park Avenue South
New York, NY 10010-1710

Contact Person
Amy S. Beacham
Telephone (Include area code)
215-239-3687

8. Complete Mailing Address of Headquarters or General Business Office of Publisher (Not printer)

Elsevier Inc., 360 Park Avenue South, New York, NY 10010-1710

9. Full Names and Complete Mailing Addresses of Publisher, Editor, and Managing Editor (Do not leave blank)

Publisher (Name and complete mailing address)

Kim Murphy, Elsevier, Inc., 1600 John F. Kennedy Blvd. Suite 1800, Philadelphia, PA 19103-2899

Editor (Name and complete mailing address)

Kerry Holland, Elsevier, Inc., 1600 John F. Kennedy Blvd. Suite 1800, Philadelphia, PA 19103-2899

Managing Editor (Name and complete mailing address)

Sarah Barth, Elsevier, Inc., 1600 John F. Kennedy Blvd. Suite 1800, Philadelphia, PA 19103-2899

10. Owner (Do not leave blank. If the publication is owned by a corporation, give the name and address of the corporation immediately followed by the names and addresses of all stockholders owning or holding 1 percent or more of the total amount of stock. If not owned by a corporation, give the names and addresses of the individual owners. If owned by a partnership or other unincorporated firm, give its name and address as well as those of each individual owner. If the publication is published by a nonprofit organization, give its name and address.)

Full Name	Complete Mailing Address
Wholly owned subsidiary of	4520 East-West Highway
Reed/Elsevier, US holdings	Bethesda, MD 20814

11. Known Bondholders, Mortgagees, and Other Security Holders Owning or Holding 1 Percent or More of Total Amount of Bonds, Mortgages, or Other Securities. If none, check box ☐ None

Full Name	Complete Mailing Address
N/A	

12. Tax Status (For completion by nonprofit organizations authorized to mail at nonprofit rates) (Check one)
The purpose, function, and nonprofit status of this organization and the exempt status for federal income tax purposes:
☐ Has Not Changed During Preceding 12 Months
☐ Has Changed During Preceding 12 Months (Publisher must submit explanation of change with this statement)

PS Form 3526, September 2007 (Page 1 of 3 (Instructions Page 3)) PSN 7530-01-000-9931 PRIVACY NOTICE: See our Privacy policy in www.usps.com

---

13. Publication Title		14. Issue Date for Circulation Data Below
Clinics in Perinatology		September 2011

15. Extent and Nature of Circulation			Average No. Copies Each Issue During Preceding 12 Months	No. Copies of Single Issue Published Nearest to Filing Date
a. Total Number of Copies (Net press run)			2686	2076
b. Paid Circulation (By Mail and Outside the Mail)	(1)	Mailed Outside-County Paid Subscriptions Stated on PS Form 3541. (Include paid distribution above nominal rate, advertiser's proof copies, and exchange copies)	1489	1338
	(2)	Mailed In-County Paid Subscriptions Stated on PS Form 3541 (Include paid distribution above nominal rate, advertiser's proof copies, and exchange copies)		
	(3)	Paid Distribution Outside the Mails Including Sales Through Dealers and Carriers, Street Vendors, Counter Sales, and Other Paid Distribution Outside USPS®	581	467
	(4)	Paid Distribution by Other Classes Mailed Through the USPS (e.g. First-Class Mail®)		
c. Total Paid Distribution (Sum of 15b (1), (2), (3), and (4))		▲	2070	1805
d. Free or Nominal Rate Distribution (By Mail and Outside the Mail)	(1)	Free or Nominal Rate Outside-County Copies Included on PS Form 3541	61	64
	(2)	Free or Nominal Rate In-County Copies Included on PS Form 3541		
	(3)	Free or Nominal Rate Copies Mailed at Other Classes Through the USPS (e.g. First-Class Mail)		
	(4)	Free or Nominal Rate Distribution Outside the Mail (Carriers or other means)		
e. Total Free or Nominal Rate Distribution (Sum of 15d (1), (2), (3) and (4))		▲	61	64
f. Total Distribution (Sum of 15c and 15e)		▲	2131	1869
g. Copies not Distributed (See instructions to publishers #4 (page #3))		▲	555	207
h. Total (Sum of 15f and g)		▲	2686	2076
i. Percent Paid (15c divided by 15f times 100)			97.14%	96.58%

16. Publication of Statement of Ownership
☐ If the publication is a general publication, publication of this statement is required. Will be printed in the **December 2011** issue of this publication. ☐ Publication not required

17. Signature and Title of Editor, Publisher, Business Manager, or Owner	Date
Amy S. Beacham – Senior Inventory Distribution Coordinator	September 16, 2011

I certify that all information furnished on this form is true and complete. I understand that anyone who furnishes false or misleading information on this form or who omits material or information requested on the form may be subject to criminal sanctions (including fines and imprisonment) and/or civil sanctions (including civil penalties).

PS Form 3526, September 2007 (Page 2 of 3)

Moving?

Make sure your subscription moves with you!

To notify us of your new address, find your **Clinics Account Number** (located on your mailing label above your name), and contact customer service at:

Email: journalscustomerservice-usa@elsevier.com

800-654-2452 (subscribers in the U.S. & Canada)
314-447-8871 (subscribers outside of the U.S. & Canada)

Fax number: 314-447-8029

Elsevier Health Sciences Division
Subscription Customer Service
3251 Riverport Lane
Maryland Heights, MO 63043